Imaging of Brain Concussion

Editors

ELIANA BONFANTE
ROY RIASCOS

NEUROIMAGING CLINICS OF NORTH AMERICA

www.neuroimaging.theclinics.com

Consulting Editor
SURESH K. MUKHERJI

February 2018 • Volume 28 • Number 1

ELSEVIER

1600 John F. Kennedy Boulevard ● Suite 1800 ● Philadelphia, Pennsylvania, 19103-2899

http://www.neuroimaging.theclinics.com

NEUROIMAGING CLINICS OF NORTH AMERICA Volume 28, Number 1
February 2018 ISSN 1052-5149, ISBN 13: 978-0-323-56990-3

Editor: John Vassallo (j.vassallo@elsevier.com)
Developmental Editor: Casey Potter

Neuroimaging Clinics of North America (ISSN 1052-5149) is published quarterly by Elsevier Inc., 360 Park Avenue South, New York, NY 10010-1710. Months of issue are February, May, August, and November. Business and editorial offices: 1600 John F. Kennedy Blvd., Suite 1800, Philadelphia, PA 19103-2899. Business and editorial offices: 6277 Sea Harbor Drive, Orlando, FL 32887-4800. Periodicals postage paid at New York, NY, and additional mailing offices. Subscription prices are USD 387 per year for US individuals, USD 622 per year for US institutions, USD 100 per year for US students and residents, USD 440 per year for Canadian individuals, USD 791 per year for Canadian institutions, USD 525 per year for international individuals, USD 791 per year for international institutions and USD 260 per year for Canadian and foreign students and residents. To receive student/resident rate, orders must be accompanied by name of affiliated institution, date of term, and the *signature* of program/residency coordinator on institution letterhead. Orders will be billed at individual rate until proof of status is received. Foreign air speed delivery is included in all *Clinics* subscription prices. All prices are subject to change without notice. POSTMASTER: Send address changes to *Neuroimaging Clinics of North America*, Elsevier Health Sciences Division, Subscription **Customer Service, 3251 Riverport Lane, Maryland Heights, MO 63043. Telephone: 1-800-654-2452 (U.S. and Canada); 314-447-8871 (outside U.S. and Canada). Fax: 314-447-8029. E-mail: journalscustomer service-usa@elsevier.com (for print support); journalsonlinesupport-usa@elsevier.com (for online support)**.

Reprints. For copies of 100 or more of articles in this publication, please contact the Commercial Reprints Department, Elsevier Inc., 360 Park Avenue South, New York, NY 10010-1710. Tel.: 212-633-3874; Fax: 212-633-3820; E-mail: reprints@elsevier.com.

Neuroimaging Clinics of North America is covered by *Excerpta Medical/EMBASE,* the RSNA Index of Imaging Literature, *MEDLINE/PubMed (Index Medicus),* MEDLINE/MEDLARS, SciSearch, Research Alert, and Neuroscience Citation Index.

PROGRAM OBJECTIVE

The goal of *Neuroimaging Clinics of North America* is to keep practicing radiologists and radiology residents up to date with current clinical practice in radiology by providing timely articles reviewing the state of the art in patient care.

TARGET AUDIENCE

Practicing radiologists, radiology residents, and other healthcare professionals who utilize neuroimaging findings to provide patient care.

LEARNING OBJECTIVES

Upon completion of this activity, participants will be able to:
1. Review imaging techniques for concussions in young athletes.
2. Discuss the uses of CT, MRI, and fMRI in concussion imaging.
3. Recognize imaging techniques for chronic concussion.

ACCREDITATION

The Elsevier Office of Continuing Medical Education (EOCME) is accredited by the Accreditation Council for Continuing Medical Education (ACCME) to provide continuing medical education for physicians.

The EOCME designates this enduring material for a maximum of 15 *AMA PRA Category 1 Credit*(s)™. Physicians should claim only the credit commensurate with the extent of their participation in the activity.

All other healthcare professionals requesting continuing education credit for this enduring material will be issued a certificate of participation.

DISCLOSURE OF CONFLICTS OF INTEREST

The EOCME assesses conflict of interest with its instructors, faculty, planners, and other individuals who are in a position to control the content of CME activities. All relevant conflicts of interest that are identified are thoroughly vetted by EOCME for fair balance, scientific objectivity, and patient care recommendations. EOCME is committed to providing its learners with CME activities that promote improvements or quality in healthcare and not a specific proprietary business or a commercial interest.

The planning committee, staff, authors and editors listed below have identified no financial relationships or relationships to products or devices they or their spouse/life partner have with commercial interest related to the content of this CME activity:

Octavio Arevalo, MD; Sonia Bermudez, MD; Eliana Bonfante, MD; Maria J. Borja, MD; Tiffany R. Chang, MD; Ruchir Chaudhari, MD; Sohae Chung, PhD; Pamela K. Douglas, PhD; Anjali Fortna; Matthew Gray, BS; Jeffrey P. Guenette, MD; James Gullo, MD; Khader M. Hasan, PhD; Zafer Keser, MD; Jared Kirkland, MD; Ivan I. Kirov, PhD; Ryan S. Kitagawa, MD; Leah Logan; Yvonne W. Lui, MD; Suresh K. Mukherji, MD, MBA, FACR; Mubashir Pervez, MD; Roy Riascos, MD; Scott Rosenthal, MS; Paul E. Schulz, MD; Karthik Subramaniam; Carlos Torres, MD, FRCPC; Juan Nicolas Useche, MD; John Vassallo; James Walroth, MD; Alexander Mark Weber, MSc, PhD; Christopher T. Whitlow, MD, PhD, MHA; Elisabeth A. Wilde, PhD; Max Wintermark, MD, MBA; Ely Wolin, MD; Carlos Zamora, MD, PhD; Jason M. Zhao, MD, PhD.

The planning committee, staff, authors and editors listed below have identified financial relationships or relationships to products or devices they or their spouse/life partner have with commercial interest related to the content of this CME activity:

David B. Douglas, MD is a consultant/advisor for, with stock ownership in, and receives royalties/patents from Springer, and has research support from and an employment affiliation with the U.S. Department of Defense.
Hudaisa Fatima, MSc has an employment affiliation with Alzheimer's Disease Clinical Core.
Theodore A. Henderson, MD, PhD has stock ownership in The Synaptic Space; Neuro-Luminance; Neuro-Laser Foundation; and Dr. Theodore Henderson, Inc.
Inga K. Koerte, MD receives royalties/patents from the National Institute of Neurological Disorders and Stroke.
Cyrus A. Raji, MD, PhD is a consultant/advisor for Brainreader ApS and Change Your Brain, Change Your Life Foundation.
Alexander Rauscher, MSc, PhD is on the speakers' bureau for Koninklijke Philips N.V.
Haris I. Sair, MD, PhD has research support from Tocagen.
Martha E. Shenton, PhD receives royalties/patents from the National Institute of Neurological Disorders and Stroke; National Institute of Mental Health; and the VA Merit Award.

UNAPPROVED/OFF-LABEL USE DISCLOSURE

The EOCME requires CME faculty to disclose to the participants:
1. When products or procedures being discussed are off-label, unlabelled, experimental, and/or investigational (not US Food and Drug Administration [FDA] approved); and
2. Any limitations on the information presented, such as data that are preliminary or that represent ongoing research, interim analyses, and/or unsupported opinions. Faculty may discuss information about pharmaceutical agents that is outside of FDA-approved labelling. This information is intended solely for CME and is not intended to promote off-label use of these

medications. If you have any questions, contact the medical affairs department of the manufacturer for the most recent prescribing information.

TO ENROLL
To enroll in the *Neuroimaging Clinics of North America* Continuing Medical Education program, call customer service at 1-800-654-2452 or sign up online at http://www.theclinics.com/home/cme. The CME program is available to subscribers for an additional annual fee of USD 235.

METHOD OF PARTICIPATION
In order to claim credit, participants must complete the following:
1. Complete enrolment as indicated above.
2. Read the activity.
3. Complete the CME Test and Evaluation. Participants must achieve a score of 70% on the test. All CME Tests and Evaluations must be completed online.

CME INQUIRIES/SPECIAL NEEDS
For all CME inquiries or special needs, please contact elsevierCME@elsevier.com.

NEUROIMAGING CLINICS OF NORTH AMERICA

THE CLINICS ARE AVAILABLE ONLINE!
Access your subscription at:
www.theclinics.com

Contributors

CONSULTING EDITOR

SURESH K. MUKHERJI, MD, MBA, FACR
Professor and Chairman, Walter F. Patenge
Endowed Chair, Department of Radiology,
Michigan State University, Chief Medical
Officer and Director of Health Care Delivery,
Michigan State University Health Team, East
Lansing, Michigan, USA

EDITORS

ELIANA BONFANTE, MD
Associate Professor, Department of Diagnostic
and Interventional Imaging, The University of
Texas Health Science Center at Houston,
McGovern Medical School, Houston, Texas,
USA

ROY RIASCOS, MD
Professor, Department of Diagnostic and
Interventional Imaging, The University of
Texas Health Science Center at Houston,
McGovern Medical School, Houston, Texas,
USA

AUTHORS

OCTAVIO AREVALO, MD
Research Fellow, Department of Diagnostic and
Interventional Imaging, The University of Texas
Health Science Center at Houston, McGovern
Medical School, Houston, Texas, USA

SONIA BERMUDEZ, MD
Associate Professor, Diagnostic and
Interventional Imaging Department, El Bosque
University, Hospital Universitario Fundacion
Santa Fe de Bogota, Bogota DC, Colombia

ELIANA BONFANTE, MD
Associate Professor, Department of Diagnostic
and Interventional Imaging, The University of
Texas Health Science Center at Houston,
McGovern Medical School, Houston, Texas, USA

MARIA J. BORJA, MD
Assistant Professor, Department of
Radiology, NYU School of Medicine,
New York, New York, USA

TIFFANY R. CHANG, MD
Assistant Professor of Neurology
and Neurosurgery, The Vivian L. Smith
Department of Neurosurgery, Mischer
Neuroscience Institute, Memorial
Hermann-Texas Medical Center, Houston,
Texas, USA

RUCHIR CHAUDHARI, MD
Clinical Fellow, Department of
Neuroradiology, Stanford University,
Stanford, California, USA

SOHAE CHUNG, PhD
Research Scientist, Department of
Radiology, NYU School of Medicine,
Center for Advanced Imaging Innovation and
Research, Bernard and Irene Schwartz Center
for Biomedical Imaging, New York, New York,
USA

DAVID B. DOUGLAS, MD
Adjunct Clinical Instructor, Department
of Neuroradiology, Stanford University,
Stanford, California, USA; Chief
of Neuroradiology, Department of Radiology,
David Grant USAF Medical Center, Travis Air
Force Base, California, USA

PAMELA K. DOUGLAS, PhD
Assistant Professor, Institute for Simulation
and Training, University of Central Florida,
Orlando, Florida, USA

HUDAISA FATIMA, MSc
Radiology Informatics and Image Processing
Laboratory (RIIPL), Division of Neuroradiology,
Department of Radiology, Wake Forest School
of Medicine, Winston-Salem, North Carolina,
USA

MATTHEW GRAY, BS
Radiology Informatics and Image Processing
Laboratory (RIIPL), Division of Neuroradiology,
Department of Radiology, Wake Forest School
of Medicine, Winston-Salem, North Carolina,
USA

JEFFREY P. GUENETTE, MD
Department of Radiology, Psychiatry
Neuroimaging Laboratory, Department of
Psychiatry, Brigham and Women's Hospital,
Harvard Medical School, Boston,
Massachusetts, USA

JAMES GULLO, MD
Resident Physician, Department of Radiology,
David Grant USAF Medical Center, Travis Air
Force Base, California, USA

KHADER M. HASAN, PhD
Associate Professor, Department of
Diagnostic and Interventional Imaging, The
University of Texas Health Science Center at
Houston, McGovern Medical School, Houston,
Texas, USA

THEODORE A. HENDERSON, MD, PhD
The Synaptic Space Inc, Neuro-Laser
Foundation, Neuro-Luminance Brain Health
Centers Inc, Dr. Theodore Henderson Inc,
Denver, Colorado, USA

ZAFER KESER, MD
Department of Neurology, The University of
Texas Health Science Center at Houston,
McGovern Medical School, Houston, Texas,
USA

JARED KIRKLAND, MD
Resident Physician, Department of Radiology,
David Grant USAF Medical Center, Travis Air
Force Base, California, USA

IVAN I. KIROV, PhD
Assistant Professor, Department of Radiology,
NYU School of Medicine, Center for Advanced
Imaging Innovation and Research, Bernard and
Irene Schwartz Center for Biomedical Imaging,
New York, New York, USA

RYAN S. KITAGAWA, MD
Assistant Professor, The Vivian L. Smith
Department of Neurosurgery, Mischer
Neuroscience Institute, Memorial
Hermann-Texas Medical Center, Houston,
Texas, USA

INGA K. KOERTE, MD
Department of Child and Adolescent Psychiatry,
Psychosomatic, and Psychotherapy,
Ludwig-Maximilians-Universität, Munich,
Germany; Psychiatry Neuroimaging Laboratory,
Department of Psychiatry, Brigham and
Women's Hospital, Massachusetts General
Hospital, Harvard Medical School, Boston,
Massachusetts, USA

YVONNE W. LUI, MD
Associate Professor, Department of Radiology,
NYU School of Medicine, New York, New York,
USA

MUBASHIR PERVEZ, MD
Assistant Professor, Department of Neurology,
University of Connecticut School of Medicine,
Hartford, Connecticut, USA

CYRUS A. RAJI, MD, PhD
Department of Radiology and Biomedical
Imaging, University of California San Francisco,
San Francisco, California, USA

ALEXANDER RAUSCHER, MSc, PhD
Assistant Professor, Department of Pediatrics,
Division of Neurology, Faculty of Medicine, The
University of British Columbia, Canada Research
Chair in Developmental Neuroimaging,
Vancouver, British Columbia, Canada

ROY RIASCOS, MD
Professor, Department of Diagnostic and
Interventional Imaging, The University of Texas
Health Science Center at Houston, McGovern
Medical School, Houston, Texas, USA

SCOTT ROSENTHAL, MS
Radiology Informatics and Image Processing
Laboratory (RIIPL), Division of Neuroradiology,
Department of Radiology, Wake Forest School of
Medicine, Winston-Salem, North Carolina, USA

HARIS I. SAIR, MD, PhD
Division of Neuroradiology, The Russell H.
Morgan Department of Radiology and
Radiological Sciences, The Johns Hopkins
University School of Medicine, Baltimore,
Maryland, USA

PAUL E. SCHULZ, MD
Department of Neurology, The University of
Texas Health Science Center at Houston,
McGovern Medical School, Houston, Texas,
USA

MARTHA E. SHENTON, PhD
Psychiatry Neuroimaging Laboratory,
Department of Psychiatry and Radiology,
Brigham and Women's Hospital, Department
of Psychiatry, Massachusetts General
Hospital, Harvard Medical School, Boston,
Massachusetts, USA; VA Boston Healthcare
System, Brockton Division, Brockton,
Massachusetts, USA

CARLOS TORRES, MD, FRCPC
Associate Professor , Department of
Radiology, University of Ottawa,
Neuroradiologist, Department of Medical
Imaging, The Ottawa Hospital, Ottawa,
Ontario, Canada

JUAN NICOLAS USECHE, MD
Chief of Neuroradiology Section, Diagnostic
and Interventional Imaging Department,
Assistant Professor, El Bosque University,
Hospital Universitario Fundacion Santa Fe de
Bogota, Bogota DC, Colombia

JAMES WALROTH, MD
Chair, Department of Radiology, David Grant
USAF Medical Center, Travis Air Force Base,
California, USA

ALEXANDER MARK WEBER, MSc, PhD
Postdoctoral Research Fellow, Department
of Pediatrics, Division of Neurology,
Faculty of Medicine, The University of British
Columbia, Vancouver, British Columbia,
Canada

CHRISTOPHER T. WHITLOW, MD, PhD, MHA
Chief of Neuroradiology and Vice Chair of
Informatics, Director, Radiology Informatics
and Image Processing Laboratory (RIIPL),
Director, CTSI Translational Imaging Program,
Director, Combined MD/PhD Program,
Department of Radiology, Department of
Biomedical Engineering, Clinical and
Translational Sciences Institute (CTSI), Wake
Forest School of Medicine, Winston-Salem,
North Carolina, USA

ELISABETH A. WILDE, PhD
Departments of Physical Medicine and
Rehabilitation, Neurology and Radiology,
Baylor College of Medicine, Michael E.
DeBakey VA Medical Center, Houston, Texas,
USA

MAX WINTERMARK, MD, MBA
Chairman, Department of Neuroradiology,
Stanford University, Stanford, California,
USA

ELY WOLIN, MD
Chief of Nuclear Medicine, Department of
Radiology, David Grant USAF Medical Center,
Travis Air Force Base, California, USA

CARLOS ZAMORA, MD, PhD
Assistant Professor, Department of
Radiology, Division of Neuroradiology, UNC
School of Medicine, The University of North
Carolina at Chapel Hill, Chapel Hill, North
Carolina, USA

JASON M. ZHAO, MD, PhD
Staff General Practitioner, Department
of Radiology, David Grant USAF
Medical Center, Travis Air Force Base,
California, USA

Contents

Traumatic brain injury (TBI) disrupts the normal function of the brain. This condition can adversely affect a person's quality of life with cognitive, behavioral, emotional, and physical symptoms that limit interpersonal, social, and occupational functioning. Although many systems exist, the simplest classification includes mild, moderate, and severe TBI depending on the nature of injury and the impact on the patient's clinical status. Patients with TBI require prompt evaluation and multidisciplinary management. Aside from the type and severity of the TBI, recovery is influenced by individual patient characteristics, social and environmental factors, and access to medical and rehabilitation services.

Conventional neuroimaging is still the mainstay in the assessment of the acute, follow-up, and chronic settings of concussion and mild traumatic brain injury (mTBI). Computed tomography (CT) is preferred for the initial assessment of acute mTBI, repeat evaluation in acute mTBI with neurologic deterioration, and cautious use in children with mTBI. Clinical rules have been developed to identify pediatric and adult patients with mTBI who can safely forego CT. MR imaging is mostly used in patients with acute mTBI when initial or follow-up CT is normal and there are persistent neurologic findings and in subacute or chronic mTBI.

In the United States alone, 1.6 to 3.8 million people have sports-related concussions yearly. The pathomechanisms of concussions may not be directly measured by conventional neuroimaging; advanced models may be needed to address the shortcomings of the current clinical protocols. Multimodal advanced imaging may provide more accurate diagnosis and predict the clinical course of concussion, assessing the efficacy of existing and emerging multifaceted therapies. In this article, the authors present an overview and pictorial display of conventional and advanced multimodal MR imaging methods that have been applied to identify the brain structures affected in traumatic brain injuries.

Conventional neuroimaging examinations are typically normal in concussed young athletes. A current focus of research is the characterization of subtle abnormalities after concussion using advanced neuroimaging techniques. These techniques have the potential to identify biomarkers of concussion. In the future, such biomarkers will likely provide important clinical information regarding the appropriate time interval before return to play, as well as the risk for prolonged postconcussive symptoms and long-term cognitive impairment. This article discusses results from advanced imaging techniques and emphasizes imaging modalities that will likely become available in the near future for the clinical evaluation of concussed young athletes.

Traumatic brain injury (TBI) is a significant problem worldwide, and neuroimaging plays a critical role in diagnosis and management. Perfusion neuroimaging techniques have been explored in TBI to determine and characterize potential perfusion neuroimaging biomarkers to aid in the diagnosis, treatment, and prognosis. In this article, computed tomography (CT) bolus perfusion, MR imaging bolus perfusion, MR imaging arterial spin labeling perfusion, and xenon CT are reviewed, with a focus on their applications in acute TBI. Future research directions are also discussed.

This article offers an overview of the application of PET and single-photon emission computed tomography brain imaging to concussion, a type of mild traumatic brain injury, and traumatic brain injury, in general. The article reviews the application of these neuronuclear imaging modalities in cross-sectional and longitudinal studies. In addition, this article frames the current literature with an overview of the basic physics and radiation exposure risks of each modality.

Myelin water imaging (MWI) provides mild traumatic brain injury (mTBI) researchers with a specific myelin biomarker and helps to further elucidate microstructural and microarchitectural changes of white matter after mTBI. Improvement of scanner hardware and software with the implementation of MWI across scanner platforms will likely result in increased research regarding the role of myelin in traumatic brain injury (TBI). Future research should include detailed investigation of myelin between 2 weeks and 2 months after injury, the use of MWI in moderate and severe TBI, and investigation of the role of myelin in chronic TBI.

Although susceptibility-weighted imaging (SWI) studies have suggested an increased number of microhemorrhages in concussion, most show no significant differences compared with controls. There have been mixed results on using SWI to predict neurologic outcomes. Drawbacks include inability to time microhemorrhages and difficulty in attributing them to the concussion. Magnetic resonance spectroscopy (MRS) in concussion can identify metabolic abnormalities, with many studies showing correlations with clinical outcome. Applications in individual patients are impeded by conflicting data and lack of consensus on an optimal protocol. Therefore, currently MRS has most utility in group-level comparisons designed to reveal the pathophysiology of concussion.

This article discusses mild traumatic brain injury (mTBI)-associated effects on brain functional connectivity assessed via resting-state functional MR imaging. Several studies have reported acute postinjury default mode network hyperconnectivity, followed by a period of decreased connectivity before later connectivity normalization in some patients. Other studies have reported mTBI-associated effects on connectivity that remain evident for up to 5 years or more. Discordance in the published literature regarding the direction of network connectivity changes (eg, increased versus decreased connectivity) may reflect differences in timing of data collection post injury, as well as the need to standardize MR imaging acquisition protocols and processing methods.

Remarkable advances have been made in the last decade in the use of diffusion MR imaging to study mild traumatic brain injury (mTBI). Diffusion imaging shows differences between patients with mTBI and healthy control groups in multiple different metrics using a variety of techniques, supporting the notion that there are microstructural injuries in patients with mTBI that radiologists have been insensitive to. Future areas of discovery in diffusion MR imaging and mTBI include larger longitudinal studies to better understand the evolution of the injury and unravel the biophysical meaning that the detected changes in diffusion MR imaging represent.

Conventional imaging findings in patients with cerebral concussion and chronic traumatic encephalopathy are absent or subtle in most cases. The most common abnormalities include cerebral volume loss, enlargement of the cavum of the septum pellucidum, cerebral microhemorrhages, and white matter signal abnormalities, all of which have poor sensitivity and specificity. Advanced imaging modalities, such as diffusion tensor imaging, blood oxygen level–dependent functional MR imaging, MR spectroscopy, perfusion imaging, PET, single-photon emission computed tomography, and magnetoencephalography detect physiologic abnormalities in symptomatic patients and, although currently in the investigation phase, may become useful in the clinical arena.

Foreword
Imaging of Brain Concussion

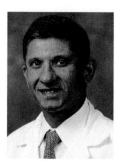

Suresh K. Mukherji, MD, MBA, FACR
Consulting Editor

Traumatic brain injury (TBI) is one of the most important health topics affecting our society. TBI touches our lives and our culture in so many ways, which include our brave military soldiers that are willing to sacrifice their health for our freedom, professional athletics, children's sports, vehicular accidents, neurorehabilitation, and the legal system. The impact of TBI was recently popularized by the movie "Concussion" that started a national dialogue on diagnosis and prevention of this "silent" disorder.

This issue of *Neuroimaging Clinics*, entitled, "Imaging of Brain Concussion," provides a comprehensive review of the state-of-the-art of the basic and advanced imaging approaches of TBI and chronic traumatic encephalopathy. Articles review the various imaging aspects of concussion, but there are also articles that address the pathophysiology and clinical impact of the

challenging topic. I want to specifically thank Drs Roy Riascos and Eliana Bonfante for accepting the challenge and creating such a wonderful issue. I also want to express my gratitude to all of the article authors for their outstanding contributions. The impact of this tremendous issue far exceeds the neuroimaging and neuroscience community and is a contribution that will directly benefit our society.

Suresh K. Mukherji, MD, MBA, FACR
Department of Radiology
Michigan State University
Michigan State University Health Team
846 Service Road
East Lansing, MI 48824, USA

E-mail address:
mukherji@rad.msu.edu

https://doi.org/10.1016/j.nic.2017.10.002
1052-5149/18/© 2017 Published by Elsevier Inc.

neuroimaging.theclinics.com

Preface

Imaging of Cerebral Concussion and Chronic Traumatic Encephalopathy

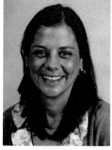 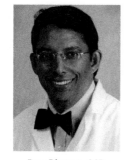

Eliana Bonfante, MD   Roy Riascos, MD

Editors

When we were invited to serve as editors of this issue on Traumatic Brain Injuries of the Head, we understood the true challenge of trying to identify an overview of this entity at a time when it has gathered significant attention from the media. Our initial effort was to meet with the different clinical and research groups that dealt with the entity to try to establish a consensus of the definition of the entity and how imaging modalities are transitioning from the research arena to clinical practice. It has definitely been a true adventure to navigate through the complex world of this entity and to find out that there is still an incredible opportunity to further investigate and apply images to the diagnosis, prognosis, and treatment follow-up of traumatic brain injury. We feel fortunate to have the collaboration of such diverse and brilliant experts participate in this issue.

Traumatic brain injury is one of the leading causes of morbidity and mortality in the United States, either as an isolated event or as associated with other injuries. The mildest presentation of the traumatic brain injury spectrum is the concussion, and its diagnosis relies on clinical grounds. Research on advanced imaging techniques has elucidated some of the complicated subjacent processes responsible for the variety of clinical outcomes seen in those patients.

This issue offers a comprehensive review of the state-of-the-art of the basic and advanced imaging approaches not only to acute but also to chronic traumatic encephalopathy. The reader will be facing a step-by-step journey over concussion imaging, going from the basics such as term definitions and its appearance in conventional computed tomography and MR imaging, to more advanced MR

Neuroimag Clin N Am 28 (2018) xvii–xviii
https://doi.org/10.1016/j.nic.2017.10.001

imaging techniques, such as perfusion-weighted imaging, diffusion-weighted imaging, diffusion tensor imaging, susceptibility-weighted imaging, and functional MR imaging. This number also includes one article dedicated to the role of single-photon emission computed tomography and PET in the evaluation of concussion patients. After a thorough literature research, authors present the most relevant imaging features of concussion, with special emphasis on those findings valuable for prognosis prediction and differential diagnosis. Furthermore, dedicated sections address the peculiarities of the imaging of concussion in young athletes and also in chronic repetitive mild brain trauma. Noteworthy, the multimodal advanced imaging assessment may provide more accurate diagnosis and predict the clinical course of concussion, assessing the efficacy of existing and emerging multifaceted therapies.

The clinical and statistical significance of many of the findings discussed in this issue are still under intense research, but it is hoped that the reader will find some useful tips in the following articles to enrich the daily practice facing concussion appraisal from the imaging point of view. As editors, we truly appreciate all the effort put forth by the authors in this publication and their commitment to excel in their articles' design and development.

The editors wish to thank Dr Octavio Arevalo for his efforts.

Eliana Bonfante, MD
Department of Diagnostic and
Interventional Imaging
The University of Texas Health
Science Center at Houston
McGovern Medical School
6431 Fannin Street, MSB 2130B
Houston, TX 77030, USA

Roy Riascos, MD
Department of Diagnostic and
Interventional Imaging
The University of Texas Health
Science Center at Houston
McGovern Medical School
6431 Fannin Street, MSB 2130B
Houston, TX 77030, USA

E-mail addresses:
Eliana.e.bonfante.mejia@uth.tmc.edu
(E. Bonfante)
Roy.F.Riascos@uth.tmc.edu (R. Riascos)

Definition of Traumatic Brain Injury, Neurosurgery, Trauma Orthopedics, Neuroimaging, Psychology, and Psychiatry in Mild Traumatic Brain Injury

Mubashir Pervez, MD[a],*, Ryan S. Kitagawa, MD[b], Tiffany R. Chang, MD[b]

KEYWORDS

- Traumatic brain injury (TBI) • Neurotrauma • Concussion • Trauma orthopedics
- Traumatic brain injury imaging • Postconcussion syndrome

KEY POINTS

- This article describes traumatic brain injury (TBI) and presents classification systems (eg, mild, moderate, or severe).
- Classification of neurotrauma orthopedics is presented.
- Initial assessment and intensive care management of TBI is discussed, including airway, breathing, circulation, and managing and stabilizing the disability (cervical and open skull fractures) come first and foremost.
- The goals of neurosurgical management are to stop the hemorrhage, remove the lesion causing mass effect, relieve high intracranial pressure, and place an invasive intracranial monitoring device, if indicated.
- Recognizing postconcussion syndrome depends on detailed history taking and focused clinical and neurologic examination.

DEFINITION OF TRAUMATIC BRAIN INJURY

Traumatic brain injury (TBI) is defined as a disruption in the normal function of the brain that can be caused by a bump, blow, or jolt to the head or a penetrating head injury.[1] The alteration in brain function caused by TBI can lead to one or more of the following symptoms:

1. Period of loss or a decreased level of consciousness;
2. Loss of memory for events immediately before (retrograde) or after the injury;
3. Neurologic deficits (weakness, loss of balance, change in vision, dyspraxia, paresis/plegia, sensory loss, aphasia, etc.); and
4. Alteration in mental state at the time of the injury (confusion, disorientation, slowed thinking, etc).[2]

Disclosure Statement: The authors have nothing to disclose.
[a] Department of Neurology, University of Connecticut School of Medicine, Jefferson Building, Suite 607, 80 Seymour Street, PO Box 5037, Hartford, CT, USA; [b] The Vivian L. Smith Department of Neurosurgery, Mischer Neuroscience Institute, Memorial Hermann-Texas Medical Center, 6431 Fannin Street MSB 7.154, Houston, TX 77030, USA
* Corresponding author.
E-mail address: mubashir.pervez@hhchealth.org

Neuroimag Clin N Am 28 (2018) 1–13
https://doi.org/10.1016/j.nic.2017.09.010
1052-5149/18/© 2017 Elsevier Inc. All rights reserved.

Classically, TBI is defined on the basis of clinical symptoms; however, modern neuroradiologic imaging techniques (eg, MR imaging–based diffusion tensor imaging) and laboratory biomarkers are being studied, which may enable a diagnosis of TBI when there is minimal or delayed clinical evidence.

SPORT-RELATED CONCUSSION

For years, the term mild TBI has been used interchangeably with sport-related concussion. More than 50 years ago, the Committee on Head Injury Nomenclature of the Congress of Neurologic Surgeons proposed a "consensus" definition of concussion, which was recognized to have a number of limitations in accounting for the common symptoms of concussion.[3,4] In the effort to update the definition, and provide recommendations for the improvement of safety of athletes who suffer concussive injuries, the international conference on concussion in sport was conducted in 2001. In 2016, the fifth International Conference on Concussion in Sport was held in which the Concussion in Sport Group updated the definition to develop further conceptual understanding of sport-related concussion. Briefly, sport-related concussion is a subset of TBI induced by biomechanical forces caused by direct blow to the head or elsewhere on the body with an impulsive force transmitted to the head. This leads to a rapid onset of short-lived impairment of neurologic function that resolves spontaneously. Sport-related concussion may result in neuropathologic changes, but the acute clinical signs and symptoms largely reflect a functional disturbance rather than a structural injury and, as such, no abnormality is seen on standard structural neuroimaging studies. Loss of consciousness may or may not be a part of a vast range of clinical signs and symptoms experienced by the athletes. Ultimately, resolution of the clinical and cognitive features typically follows a sequential course. However, in some cases symptoms may be prolonged.[5]

EPIDEMIOLOGY

TBI is a major cause of disability and death, especially in young adults, and contributes to approximately 30% of all injury deaths.[6] More than 2.5 million emergency department visits, hospitalizations, and deaths in United States are associated with TBI. The rate of TBI has also increased over the past decade from 521.0 per 100,000 in 2001 to a rate of 823.7 per 100,000 in 2010.[7]

Brain injury occurs in all age groups; however, mortality is highest in the population older than 65 years of age. Overall rates of TBI in men are 29% higher than in women. TBI-related deaths in children 0 to 4 years are primarily associated with assault (42.9%) and motor vehicle accidents (29.2%). Motor vehicle traffic crashes account for a majority of TBI-related deaths (55.8%) in youth 5 to 14 years and almost one-half (47.4%) in young adults 15 to 24 years. Falls account for the majority (54.4%) of TBI-related deaths in adults 65 years of age and older.[7]

CLASSIFICATION OF TRAUMATIC BRAIN INJURY

TBI can be classified in a number of ways but traditionally the classification is based on:

1. Clinical severity and duration of symptoms,[8] and
2. Characteristics and location of the injury.[9]

Clinical Severity and Duration of Symptoms

Concussion or cerebral contusion

- No loss of consciousness or loss of consciousness for less than 6 hours.
- No or mild memory deficit.
- Minutes to hours of posttraumatic amnesia.
- No or mild motor deficits.

Diffuse axonal injury

Mild
- Loss of consciousness lasting for 6 to 24 hours.
- Mild to moderate memory deficit.
- Hours of posttraumatic amnesia.
- Mild motor deficit.

Moderate
- Loss of consciousness for more than 24 hours.
- Moderate memory deficit.
- Days of posttraumatic amnesia.
- Moderate motor deficit.

Severe
- Loss of consciousness lasting for days to weeks.
- Severe memory deficit.
- Weeks of posttraumatic amnesia.
- Severe motor deficit.

Acceleration–deceleration injuries of the head cause the stretching, shearing, and disruption of the reticular activating system and has been proposed to be the cause of the loss of consciousness.

Table 1
Characteristics of primary and secondary TBI

	Primary TBI	Secondary TBI
Time of occurrence	Immediately at the time of impact	Hours to days after impact
Mechanism	Direct mechanical trauma	Complications initiated by the primary injury such as inflammation, cell receptor-mediated dysfunction, free radical and oxidative damage, and calcium or other ion-mediated cell damage.

Abbreviation: TBI, traumatic brain injury.

Characteristics and Location of Injury

A. Primary or secondary TBI (**Table 1**).
B. Local or diffuse TBI.

TBI can be classified by the location and the characteristic of the injury as examined on the computed tomography (CT) scan or MR imaging scan. These lesions may be focal brain lesions or diffuse injury involving multiple regions of the brain.[9]

a. Cerebral contusion.
b. Subdural hematoma.
c. Epidural hematoma.
d. Traumatic subarachnoid hemorrhage.
e. Shearing injury and diffuse axonal injury (DAI).

Cerebral contusion
Cerebral contusions are focal or diffuse parenchymal hemorrhages typically seen in locations where the brain collides with the adjacent irregular inner table of the skull (**Figs. 1** and **2**). The inferior frontal and temporal regions are the most common locations. Contusions can also occur because of the depressed skull fractures lacerating the brain tissue. These lesions may appear as coup and counter-coup lesions affecting the brain at the site of blow to the head and area opposite to that, respectively. The overlying layers of the meninges may or may not stay intact. These lesions may expand in volume naturally or due to coagulopathy and appear as different densities on CT scans and MR imaging.[10]

Subdural hematoma
Injury to the head causing hemorrhage between the brain and the dura owing to tearing of the bridging veins or rupture of cortical arteries leads to the formation of subdural hematomas (**Figs. 3** and **4**). The blood may accumulate in the lateral

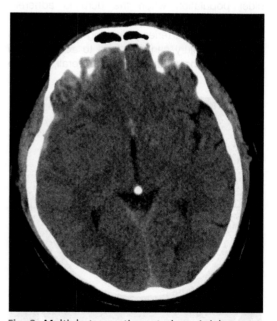

Fig. 1. Traumatic focal contusion noted on the noncontrast computed tomography of the head axial images in the right temporal lobe.

Fig. 2. Multiple traumatic contusions. Axial noncontrast computed tomography scan of the head demonstrates multiple lesions/contusions noted in bilateral frontal lobe with a right-sided acute-on-chronic traumatic subdural hematoma with mass effect.

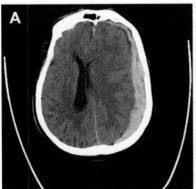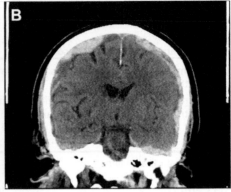

Fig. 3. (A) Computed tomography (CT) scan of the head. Axial noncontrast image demonstrates an acute traumatic subdural hematoma on the left side causing mass effect and left to right midline shift and subfalcine herniation. (B) Noncontrast CT scan of the head coronal image shows bilateral acute traumatic subdural hematoma.

aspects of the frontal, parietal, occipital, or temporal regions of the brain. Falcine and tentorial subdural hematomas are noted at the medial aspect of the frontal and cerebellar region, respectively. Risk factors for subdural hematoma are advanced age, alcohol use, and coagulopathy (Table 2).[11–14]

Epidural hematoma
Bleeding within the space between the dura and the skull leads to the accumulation of epidural hematoma. It is observed in roughly 2% to 5% of patients with TBI and is more common in the younger population; however, it can also be seen in the older population when the dura is adherent the skull. The most common cause is tearing of the meningeal arteries. Bleeding secondary to dural sinus injury can also lead to accumulation of blood in the epidural space. Overall, 75% to

80% of epidural hematomas are associated with skull fractures.[15] Epidural hematomas are typically biconvex in shape and can cause a mass effect with herniation (Fig. 5). They are usually limited by cranial sutures, but not by venous sinuses. Epidural hematomas are unilateral in more than 95% of cases; however, bilateral or multiple epidural hematomas are possible. More than 95% are supratentorial (temporoparietal, 60%; frontal, 20%; parietooccipital, 20%).[16]

Classically, the initial symptom is loss of consciousness caused by the initial impact, followed by a lucid interval. Subsequently, if the hematoma continues to expand, the patient develops focal neurologic deficits that progresses to coma. If the expanding hematoma is not managed appropriately, cerebral herniation can result. This expansion is faster and more hazardous in epidural

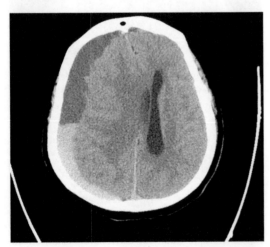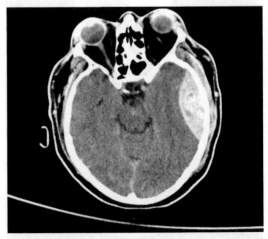

Fig. 4. Computed tomography scan of the head. Noncontrast axial image shows a right-sided acute-on-chronic subdural hematoma with mass effect and subfalcine herniation.

Fig. 5. Noncontrast computed tomography scan of the head shows an acute traumatic epidural hematoma on the left temporal region causing mass effect and transtentorial herniation.

Table 2
Symptoms onset, risk factors, and presenting symptoms of acute and chronic subdural hematoma

	Acute Subdural Hematoma	Chronic Subdural Hematoma
Symptom onset	Within 72 h	Mostly after 21 d
Risk factors	Fall Assault Trauma	Bleeding disorder Alcoholism Over drainage of ventriculoperitoneal shunt Cerebral atrophy Antiplatelet and anticoagulants
Common presenting symptoms	Seizures Acute onset headache Motor deficit Aphasia Difficulty with gait or balance	Decreased level of consciousness Headache Difficulty with gait or balance Cognitive dysfunction or memory loss Personality change Motor deficit Aphasia

hematomas because the bleed is often arterial and can lead to high mortality rates if left untreated.

Traumatic subarachnoid hemorrhage
Traumatic subarachnoid hemorrhage is a common phenomenon after TBI. It is present in around 35% of head injury patients. Hemorrhage is mostly seen in the cerebral sulci; however, it may be seen in the Sylvian fissure and basal cisterns, and is mostly associated with tearing of the pial vessels (Fig. 6).[17] CT scan of the head is considered to be a reliable tool for identifying traumatic subarachnoid hemorrhage in patients with a head injury.

Complications, including hydrocephalus and cerebral vasospasm, have been identified with

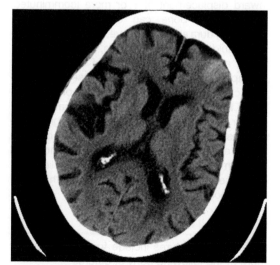

Fig. 6. Computed tomography of the head. Axial image shows left frontal trace traumatic subarachnoid hemorrhage.

traumatic subarachnoid hemorrhage and should be considered while managing patients with traumatic subarachnoid hemorrhage. However, these complications are more commonly seen as a complication of aneurysmal subarachnoid hemorrhage.[18]

Shearing injury and diffuse axonal injury
DAI is a severe form of TBI leading to loss of consciousness or coma lasting more than 6 hours. It is further classified into mild, moderate, and severe DAI, depending on the duration of coma.[8]

- Mild DAI: 6 to 24 hours.
- Moderate DAI: greater than 24 hours.
- Severe DAI: days to weeks.

DAI is the result of traumatic shearing forces that occur when the head is rapidly accelerated or decelerated. These forces cause edema at the cellular level and shearing of axons in severe cases. Misalignment of cytoskeletal elements after a stretch injury can lead to tearing of the axon and death of the neuron. The axonal transport continues up to the point of the break in the cytoskeleton, leading to a buildup of transport products and local swelling.[19] At the site of the break in the cytoskeleton, the axon can draw back toward the cell body and form a bulb. This bulb is called a retraction ball,[20] the hallmark of DAI. When the axon is transected, the axon distal to the break degenerates, leading to Wallerian degeneration.[21]

The most common sites of DAI are:

- Parasagittal white matter,
- Periventricular region,
- Internal capsule,
- Corpus collosum,

- Pons, and
- Dorsolateral midbrain.

Although a noncontrast CT scan is typically the initial imaging for all patients with TBI, the sensitivity of a CT scan is low for detecting DAI. MR imaging, especially the gradient echo and fluid attenuation inversion recovery sequences, are the imaging modalities of choice in cases of DAI with and without hemorrhage, respectively (Fig. 7).

TRAUMA ORTHOPEDICS

TBI may be associated with linear, depressed, and basilar skull fractures. The severity of injury and type of fracture are associated with the risk of underlying parenchymal injury. Open skull fractures are more complicated than closed ones because of the direct contact between the environment and brain parenchyma, increasing the risk of infection.

Skull fractures may be divided into:

- Linear skull fracture,
- Depressed skull fracture,
- Basilar skull fracture, and
- Penetrating skull fracture.

Linear Skull Fracture

Linear skull fractures occur mostly in the temporoparietal, frontal, and occipital regions (Fig. 8). The majority of linear fractures are benign and have minimal clinical significance. However, if the fracture line

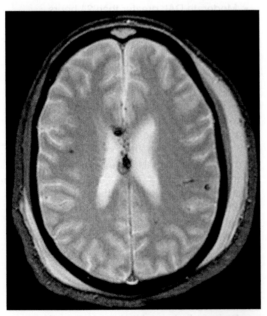

Fig. 7. MR imaging of the brain. Axial images shows areas of extensive axonal brain injury mainly in the corpus collosum area.

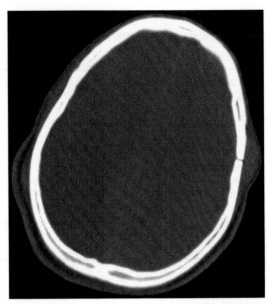

Fig. 8. Computed tomography scan of the head. Axial images showing linear fracture of the left parietal bone extending into the coronal sutures.

crosses the middle meningeal groove, dural venous sinuses, or temporal bone, the risk of affecting or damaging the vascular structures and causing secondary extraaxial hematomas is present.

Most linear skull fractures are managed conservatively. If the linear skull fracture is associated with underlying hemorrhage or diastasis of the suture lines, neurosurgical intervention may be required.

Depressed Skull Fracture

Inward displacement of 1 or more (comminuted) fragments of bone can cause injury to the underlying dura and brain tissue, leading to cerebrospinal fluid (CSF) leak, infection, seizures, hemorrhage, and ultimately death if not treated in time and appropriately (Fig. 9).[22] Depressed skull fractures can be open or closed depending on the integrity of the overlying skin; if open, the patient is at greater risk for complications. Neurosurgical procedures, including surgical exploration, debridement, elevation of bone fragments, and dural repair, may be required to prevent complications. Depressed skull fractures also increased the risk of dural venous thrombosis and laceration.[23–25]

Basilar Skull Fracture

Basilar skull fractures include fractures of one or more of the following bony structures[26]:

- Cribriform plate of the ethmoid bone,
- Orbital plate of the frontal bone,

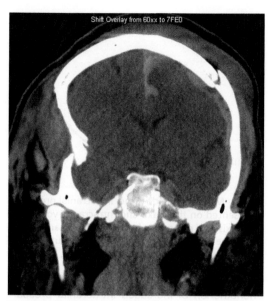

Fig. 9. Computed tomography scan of the head. Coronal image shows depressed fracture of the right temporal and sphenoid bones resulting in compression of the right temporal lobe with uncal herniation.

- Petrous and squamous portion of the temporal bone,
- Sphenoid bone, and
- Occipital bone.

The following clinical signs are highly predictive of basilar skull fractures. These clinical signs may not appear immediately after the trauma, and may take hours to days to manifest.[27]

- Retroauricular or mastoid ecchymosis (Battle sign),
- Periorbital ecchymosis (Raccoon eye),
- Rhinorrhea,
- Otorrhea,
- Hemotympanum and tympanic membrane perforation,
- Peripheral facial nerve weakness,
- Anosmia, and
- Hearing loss.

Traumatic carotid cavernous fistula is also a rare but important complication of basilar skull fractures.[28] Early neurosurgical consultation, extraaxial hematoma evacuation, CSF leak repair, antibiotics, and anticonvulsants are the mainstay treatments, depending on the location of the fracture and the complications associated with it.

Penetrating Skull Fracture

Penetrating skull fractures occur as a result of gunshot wounds, stab wounds, and blast injuries (Fig. 10). Generally these cases carry a worse

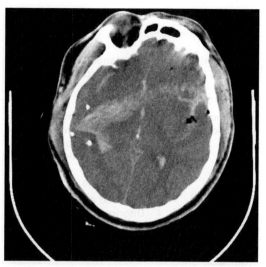

Fig. 10. Computed tomography scan of the head. Axial images shows generalized cerebral edema, mass effect, intraventricular hemorrhage, and bilateral hemispheric intraparenchymal hemorrhage secondary to gunshot wound to the head. Bullet pellet can be visualized as a hyperdense foreign object in the right frontoparietal region.

prognosis. Several CT scan findings have been documented to be associated with worse outcome. These include bihemispheric lesions, multilobar injuries, intraventricular hemorrhage, uncal herniation, and subarachnoid hemorrhage.[29]

INITIAL ASSESSMENT, AND NEUROSURGICAL AND NEUROINTENSIVE CARE MANAGEMENT

The initial assessment of a patient with TBI comprises resuscitation measures, history taking, and neurologic examination. As with all emergent cases, airway, breathing, circulation, and managing and stabilizing the disability (cervical and open skull fractures) come first and foremost.

At this time, assessing the severity of neurologic compromise secondary to the TBI is important to decide whether the patient needs emergent neurosurgical procedures such as intracranial pressure monitoring, CSF diversion, craniotomy or craniectomy, burr holes, debridement, or evacuation of mass lesions. The assessment of severity depends on clinical examination, assessment tools like the Glasgow Coma Scale, and imaging studies (Table 3).

ADMISSION CRITERIA

Admission criteria to the hospital and intensive care unit varies from hospital to hospital, but

Table 3
Glasgow Coma Scale

Eye opening (E)	4 – Spontaneously
	3 – To verbal commands
	2 – To pain
	1 – No response
Best motor response (M)	6 – Obeys commands
	5 – Localizes to pain
	4 – Flexion withdrawal
	3 – Abnormal flexion
	2 – Extension
	1 – No response
Best verbal response (V)	5 – Oriented and converses
	4 – Disoriented and converses
	3 – Inappropriate words
	2 – Incomprehensible sounds
	1 – No response

Adapted from Teasdale G, Jennett B. Assessment of coma and impaired consciousness. A practical scale. Lancet 1974;2(7872):81–4; with permission.

generally patients will require monitoring if presenting with the following:

- Low Glasgow Coma Scale score, confusion, or depressed level of consciousness;
- Focal neurologic signs on examination;
- Seizures;
- Drug or alcohol abuse;
- Intracranial bleeding;
- Depressed fractures;
- Active antiplatelet and anticoagulation with concerns of worsening hemorrhage;
- Multiple medical conditions (cardiac, hepatic, renal compromise or failure); and
- Unsafe to be discharged home.

MANAGEMENT OF INCREASED INTRACRANIAL PRESSURE

The human brain is enclosed in a fixed cranium composed of CSF, brain parenchyma, and blood. The presence of a space-occupying lesion or an increase in volume of one these compartments, without compensatory changes in another compartment, ultimately leads to increased intracranial pressure (Fig. 11). This hypothesis was first introduced in the Monro-Kellie doctrine.[30]

Depressed level of alertness or consciousness, confusion, disorientation, vision changes, diplopia, headache, nausea, and vomiting are signs and symptoms of increased intracranial pressure. If the intracranial pressure continues to increase, the patient may present with signs of Cushing triad (hypertension, bradycardia, and irregular respirations). This well-known

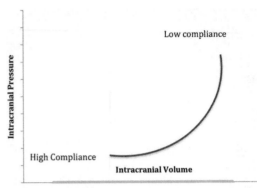

Fig. 11. Monro-Kellie doctrine. Intracranial pressure is represented on the *y*-axis and intracranial volume on the *x*-axis. The presence of a mass lesion or an increase in volume of 1 these compartments, without compensatory changes in another compartment, ultimately leads to increased intracranial pressure.

phenomenon of increased intracranial pressure ultimately leads to cerebral herniation and death. Different herniation syndromes are described in Table 4.

The stepwise critical care management of patient with traumatic brain injuries with worsening intracranial pressure may include the following[31–49]:

- Secure airway, breathing, and maintain adequate circulation and cerebral perfusion pressure;
- Elevation of head position;
- Transient hyperventilation;
- Adequate sedation;
- Hyperosmolar therapy;
- Anticonvulsant therapy;
- Intracranial monitor placement;
- Decompressive neurosurgery;
- Barbiturates; and
- Hypothermia (Fig. 12).

Corticosteroids are associated with an increased rate of death in patients who were given a high dose of steroids during the first week after TBI. They are also known to increase the risk of infection, hyperglycemia, impaired wound healing, and delirium if used in high doses for longer time intervals.[50] Routine use of steroids in the setting of TBI is therefore not recommended.

NEUROSURGICAL INTERVENTIONS IN TRAUMATIC BRAIN INJURY

The goals of neurosurgical management in patients with TBI are to:

- Stop the hemorrhage,
- Remove the lesion causing mass effect,

Table 4
Location and characteristics of intracranial herniation syndromes

Location of Herniation	Characteristic	Clinical Syndrome
Subfalcine	Displacement of the brain (typically the cingulate gyrus) beneath the free edge of the falx cerebri owing to increased intracranial pressure	• Somnolence • Contralateral hydrocephalus • ACA compression causing contralateral leg weakness
Uncal (transtentorial)	The innermost part of the temporal lobe, the uncus, can be squeezed so much that it moves toward the tentorium and puts pressure on the brainstem, most notably the midbrain	• Somnolence • Anisocoria to ipsilateral 'blown pupil' • Midbrain compression • PCA compression • Duret hemorrhages • Extensive midline shift owing to mass effect, resulting in indentation in the contralateral cerebral crus by the tentorium cerebelli. This has also been referred to as the Kernohan-Woltman notch phenomenon.
Upward herniation (upward transtentorial)	Space-occupying lesions in the posterior cranial fossa cause superior displacement of superior parts of the cerebellum through the tentorial notch.	• Somnolence • Ischemia in the PCA and SCA territory • Bilateral 'blown' pupil
Tonsillar	Inferior descent of the cerebellar tonsils below the foramen magnum.	• Somnolence • Quadriparesis • Cardiac arrhythmias • Respiratory failure

Abbreviations: ACA, anterior cerebral artery; PCA, posterior cerebral artery; SCA, superior cerebellar artery.

Data from Laine FJ, Shedden AI, Dunn MM, et al. Acquired intracranial herniations: MR imaging findings. Am J Roentgenol 1995;165(4):967–73.

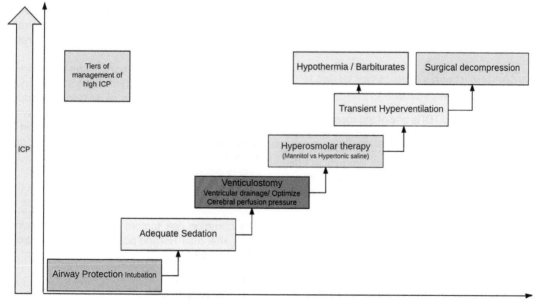

Fig. 12. Tiers of management of high intracranial pressure (ICP) in a patient with traumatic brain injury.

- Relieve high intracranial pressure, and
- Invasive intracranial monitoring device placement, if indicated.

Surgical removal of a portion of the skull, known as decompressive craniectomy, has been studied for the purpose of relieving increased intracranial pressure and improved outcomes in TBI. DECRA (Decompressive Craniectomy in Diffuse Traumatic Brain Injury) and RESCUEicp (Randomised Evaluation of Surgery with Craniectomy for Uncontrollable Elevation of Intracranial Pressure) are 2 recent randomized controlled trials of surgical decompression in TBI. In 2011, the DECRA study showed that there was no benefit from bifrontal surgical decompressive craniectomy to reduce intracranial pressure,[45] although the generalizability of the negative results and the definition of refractory intracranial pressure were the major points that were called into question. Later in 2016, the RESCUEicp[51] trial compared decompressive surgery with medical management in patients with TBI and increased intracranial pressure. At 6 months, surgery was associated with lower mortality, higher vegetative state, higher lower severe disability, and higher upper severe disability rates, with similar rates of moderate disability and good recovery. Intracranial pressure was better controlled in the surgical group. The study concluded that decompressive craniectomy is a life-saving intervention for refractory intracranial hypertension in patients with TBI.

It is important to engage the patient's family and surrogates in surgical decision making in light of the patient's previously expressed wishes. At this time, the care of patients with TBI should be individualized and further randomized trials are needed to clarify optimal surgical management in specific patient populations.

PSYCHOLOGY AND PSYCHIATRY IN MILD TRAUMATIC BRAIN INJURY

Concussion or mild TBI is one of the most common forms of TBI. The majority of individuals who sustain such injuries are young adults. Initially, mild TBI was considered to be a mild, insignificant disorder. However, this disease has now been shown to be a neuropathologic disorder with considerable neurophysiologic consequences requiring formal evaluation and management.[52]

Individuals sustaining mild head injuries often complain of a number of physical, cognitive, and emotional/behavioral symptoms referred to as postconcussion symptoms. These symptoms can persist from months to years after injury and may even cause permanent disability (Table 5).[53]

Table 5
Common symptoms of mild TBI and postconcussion syndrome

Physical symptoms	Headache Dizziness Fatigue Visual symptoms Light sensitivity Noise sensitivity
Cognitive symptoms	Memory deficit Attention and concentration deficit Executive function deficit Retrograde or anterograde amnesia
Emotional or psychological symptoms	Mood disorder Depression Anxiety

There are an estimated 1.6 to 3.8 million sport-related concussions annually in the United States. Although the majority of patients who sustain a concussion will reach full neurologic recovery within 1 to 2 weeks, about 15% to 20% will demonstrate persistent signs and symptoms lasting more than 3 weeks.[54]

Dizziness, insomnia, fatigue, mood disorders, and an inability to concentrate with or without anxiety and depression are common symptoms of postconcussion syndrome. The phenomenon is more commonly witnessed in patients with a prior history of mood or psychiatric disorders. The general hypothesis is that the mechanisms behind symptoms of postconcussion syndrome are composed of complex processes at the molecular level, leading to alterations in cell membrane permeability, ion transport regulation, neurotransmitter release, cellular metabolism, and cerebral blood flow.[55]

The severity of the postconcussive symptoms is not consistently correlated with the nature, intensity, or severity of the initial brain injury. Cognitive impairment is one of the most commonly reported symptoms in this patient population including short- or long-term memory impairment, difficulty with maintaining attention, decreased concentration, language disorders, and alteration in personality.

Risk Factors for Postconcussion Syndrome

The common risk factors associated with symptoms after mild TBI and postconcussion syndrome are as follows[56–59]:

- Younger age,
- Female gender,
- Prior concussion history,

- Baseline learning disabilities,
- History of migraine headaches, and
- History of psychological or mood disorders.

Recognizing postconcussion syndrome depends on detailed history taking and a focused clinical and neurologic examination. The graded treadmill test may be used to quantify the degree of symptoms of postconcussion syndrome.[60,61]

Chronic Traumatic Encephalopathy

Chronic traumatic encephalopathy (CTE) is a progressive neurodegenerative condition associated with repetitive head trauma. CTE is considered one of the tauopathies, marked by an accumulation of hyperphosphorylated tau protein, leading to neuronal destruction and accompanying symptoms. CTE was first described in 1928, when Dr Harrison Martland described a group of boxers as having "punch drunk syndrome."[62,63] Over the next 75 years, several researchers reported similar findings in boxers and victims of brain trauma, but fewer than 50 cases were confirmed. In 2005, a pathologist named Bennet Omalu published the first evidence of CTE in an American football player. Later, among the 202 deceased former players of American football who were part of a brain donation program, a high proportion (approximately 177) was neuropathologically diagnosed with CTE. The one thing in common in most of the cases with CTE is a history of repetitive head impacts. Behavioral, mood, cognitive, and motor symptoms are identified as common symptoms associated with mild or severe CTE.[64] The concept and studies on CTE are still in the initial phases. Once a combination of clinical diagnostic criteria and accurate biomarkers is validated, future research of the risk factors, clinical course, prevention, and treatment will be the target.[65,66]

Management Strategies for Postconcussion Syndrome

Depending on the intensity, duration, and nature of symptoms the patient might benefit from:

- Physical and cognitive rest,
- School accommodations,
- Aerobic exercise programs for adolescent and adult athletes,
- Vestibular rehabilitation programs,
- Vision therapy programs,
- Balance and gaze stabilization exercises,
- Cervical spine manual therapy, and
- Head–neck proprioception retraining.

SUMMARY

- TBI causes disruption of the normal brain function affecting cognition, behavioral and emotional states, and physical symptoms.
- Early recognition by clinical and radiographic testing is critical for the diagnosis and management of TBI.
- Multidisciplinary management by emergency physicians, neurologists, neurointensivists, and neurosurgeons is important for the management of complications of TBI.
- Early neurosurgical assessment for neurosurgical intervention is crucial.
- Mood disorders like anxiety and depression are frequent psychiatric complications of TBI

REFERENCES

1. Faul M, Xu L, Wald MM, et al. Traumatic brain injury in the United States: emergency department visits, hospitalizations, and deaths. Centers Dis Control Prev Natl Cent Inj Prev Control 2010:891–904.
2. Menon DK, Schwab K. Position statement: definition of traumatic brain injury. Arch Phys Med Rehabil 2010;91(11):1637–40.
3. Congress of Neurological Surgeons. Committee on head injury nomenclature: glossary of head injury. Clin Neurosurg 1966;12:386–94, 3.
4. Johnston K, McCrory P, Mohtadi N, et al. Evidence based review of sport related concussion: clinical science. Clin J Sport Med 2001;11:150–60.
5. McCrory P, Meeuwisse W, Dvorak J, et al. Consensus statement on concussion in sport—the 5th international conference on concussion in sport held in Berlin, October 2016. Br J Sports Med 2017. https://doi.org/10.1136/bjsports-2017-097699.
6. Marr A, Coronado V. Central nervous system injury surveillance data submission standards – 2002. Atlanta (GA): Centers for Disease Control and Prevention, National Center for Injury Prevention and Control; 2004.
7. Frieden TR, Houry D, Baldwin G. Traumatic brain injury in the United States: epidemiology and rehabilitation 2015. doi:10.3171/2009.10.JNS091500.
8. Gennarelli TA. Cerebral concussion and diffuse brain lesions. In: Cooper PR, editor. Head lesion. 3rd edition. Baltimore (MD): Williams & Wilkins; 1993. p. 137–58.
9. Marshall LF, Marshall SB, Klauber MR, et al. The diagnosis of head injury requires a classification based on computed axial tomography. J Neurotrauma 1992; 9(Suppl 1):S287–92.
10. Stein S, Spettell C, Young G, et al. Delayed and progressive brain injury in closed-head trauma: radiological demonstration. Neurosurgery 1993;32(1):25–30.

11. Teale EA, Iliffe S, Young JB. Subdural haematoma in the elderly. BMJ 2014;348:g1682.

12. Adhiyaman V, Asghar M, Ganeshram K, et al. Chronic subdural haematoma in the elderly. Postgrad Med J 2002;78(916):71.

13. Sim Y-W, Min K-S, Lee M-S, et al. Recent changes in risk factors of chronic subdural hematoma. J Korean Neurosurg Soc 2012;52(3):234–9.

14. Rust T, Kiemer N, Erasmus A. Chronic subdural haematomas and anticoagulation or anti-thrombotic therapy. J Clin Neurosci 2006;13(8):823–7.

15. Irie F, Le Brocque R, Kenardy J, et al. Epidemiology of traumatic epidural hematoma in young age. J Trauma 2011;71(4):847–53.

16. Takeuchi S, Wada K, Takasato Y, et al. Traumatic hematoma of the posterior fossa. Acta Neurochir Suppl 2013;118:135–8.

17. Wu Z, Li S, Lei J, et al. Evaluation of traumatic subarachnoid hemorrhage using susceptibility-weighted imaging. AJNR Am J Neuroradiol 2010; 31(7):1302–10.

18. Oertel M, Boscardin WJ, Obrist WD, et al. Posttraumatic vasospasm: the epidemiology, severity, and time course of an underestimated phenomenon: a prospective study performed in 299 patients. J Neurosurg 2005;103(5):812–24.

19. Staal JA, Dickson TC, Chung RS, et al. Cyclosporin-A treatment attenuates delayed cytoskeletal alterations and secondary axotomy following mild axonal stretch injury. Dev Neurobiol 2007;67(14):1831–42.

20. Wasserman JR, Feldman JS, Koenigsberg RA. Diffuse axonal injury. eMedicine.com. doi:10.1007/3-540-27660-2_104.

21. LoPachin RM, Lehning EJ. Mechanism of calcium entry during axon injury and degeneration. Toxicol Appl Pharmacol 1997;143(2):233–44.

22. Braakman R. Depressed skull fracture: data, treatment, and follow-up in 225 consecutive cases. J Neurol Neurosurg Psychiatry 1972;35(3):395–402.

23. Delgado Almandoz JE, Kelly HR, Schaefer PW, et al. Prevalence of traumatic dural venous sinus thrombosis in high-risk acute blunt head trauma patients evaluated with multidetector CT venography. Radiology 2010;255(2):570–7.

24. Zhao X, Rizzo A, Malek B, et al. Basilar skull fracture: a risk factor for transverse/sigmoid venous sinus obstruction. J Neurotrauma 2008;25(2):104–11.

25. Miller JD, Jennett WB. Complications of depressed skull fracture. Lancet 1968;292(7576):991–5.

26. Golfinos JG, Cooper PR. Skull fracture and post-traumatic cerebrospinal fluid fistula. In: Cooper PR, Golfinos JG, editors. Head Injury. 4th edition. New York: McGraw-Hill; 2000. p. 155.

27. Tubbs RS, Shoja MM, Loukas M, et al. William Henry Battle and Battle's sign: mastoid ecchymosis as an indicator of basilar skull fracture. J Neurosurg 2010;112(1):186–8.

28. Fattahi TT, Brandt MT, Jenkins WS, et al. Traumatic carotid-cavernous fistula: pathophysiology and treatment. J Craniofac Surg 2003;14(2):240–6.

29. Esposito DP, Walker JB. Contemporary management of penetrating brain injury. Neurosurg Q 2009;19(4):249–54.

30. Mokri B. The Monro-Kellie hypothesis: applications in CSF volume depletion. Neurology 2001;56(12):1746–8.

31. Davis DP. Early ventilation in traumatic brain injury. Resuscitation 2008;76(3):333–40.

32. Moppett IK. Traumatic brain injury: assessment, resuscitation and early management. Br J Anaesth 2007;99(1):18–31.

33. John R, Appleby I. Traumatic brain injury: initial resuscitation and transfer. Anaesth Intensive Care Med 2014;15(4):161–3.

34. Durward QJ, Amacher AL, Del Maestro RF, et al. Cerebral and cardiovascular responses to changes in head elevation in patients with intracranial hypertension. J Neurosurg 1983;59(6):938–44.

35. Bouma GJ, Muizelaar JP. Cerebral blood flow, cerebral blood volume, and cerebrovascular reactivity after severe head injury. J Neurotrauma 1992; 9(Suppl 1):S333–48. Available at: http://www.ncbi.nlm.nih.gov/pubmed/1588625.

36. Yundt KD, Diringer MN. The use of hyperventilation and its impact on cerebral ischemia in the treatment of traumatic brain injury. Crit Care Clin 1997;13(1):163–84.

37. Coles JP, Fryer TD, Coleman MR, et al. Hyperventilation following head injury: effect on ischemic burden and cerebral oxidative metabolism. Crit Care Med 2007;35(2):568–78.

38. Oddo M, Crippa IA, Mehta S, et al. Optimizing sedation in patients with acute brain injury. Crit Care 2016;20(1):128.

39. Cooper DJ, Myles PS, McDermott FT, et al. Prehospital hypertonic saline resuscitation of patients with hypotension and severe traumatic brain injury: a randomized controlled trial. JAMA 2004;291(11):1350–7.

40. White H, Cook D, Venkatesh B. The use of hypertonic saline for treating intracranial hypertension after traumatic brain injury. Anesth Analg 2006;102(6):1836–46.

41. Temkin NR, Dikmen SS, Winn HR. Management of head injury. Posttraumatic seizures. Neurosurg Clin N Am 1991;2(2):425–35. Available at: http://www.ncbi.nlm.nih.gov/htbin-post/Entrez/query?db=m&form=6&dopt=r&uid=1821751.

42. Szaflarski JP, Sangha KS, Lindsell CJ, et al. Prospective, randomized, single-blinded comparative trial of intravenous levetiracetam versus phenytoin for seizure prophylaxis. Neurocrit Care 2010;12(2):165–72.

43. Chesnut RM, Temkin N, Carney N, et al. A trial of intracranial-pressure monitoring in traumatic brain injury. N Engl J Med 2012;367(26):2471–81.

44. Alali AS, Fowler RA, Mainprize TG, et al. Intracranial pressure monitoring in severe traumatic brain injury: results from the American College of Surgeons Trauma Quality Improvement Program. J Neurotrauma 2013;30(20):1737–46.

45. Cooper DJ, Rosenfeld JV, Murray L, et al. Decompressive craniectomy in diffuse traumatic brain injury. N Engl J Med 2011;364(16):1493–502.

46. Shutter LA, Timmons SD. Intracranial pressure rescued by decompressive surgery after traumatic brain injury. N Engl J Med 2016;375(12):1183–4.

47. Roberts I, Sydenham E. Barbiturates for acute traumatic brain injury. Cochrane Database Syst Rev 2012;(12):CD000033.

48. Fox JL, Vu EN, Doyle-Waters M, et al. Prophylactic hypothermia for traumatic brain injury: a quantitative systematic review. CJEM 2010;12(4):355–64.

49. Carney N, Totten AM, O'Reilly C, et al. Guidelines for the management of severe traumatic brain injury, fourth edition. Neurosurgery 2017;80(1):6–15.

50. Roberts I, Yates D, Sandercock P, et al. Effect of intravenous corticosteroids on death within 14 days in 10 008 adults with clinically significant head injury (MRC CRASH trial): randomised placebo-controlled trial. Lancet 2004;364(9442):1321–8.

51. Hutchinson PJ, Kolias AG, Timofeev IS, et al. Trial of decompressive craniectomy for traumatic intracranial hypertension. N Engl J Med 2016;375(12):1119–30.

52. Dikmen SS, Levin HS. Methodological issues in the study of mild head injury. J Head Trauma Rehabil 1993;8(3):30–7.

53. Brown SJ, Fann JR, Grant I. Postconcussional disorder: time to acknowledge a common source of neurobehavioral morbidity. J Neuropsychiatry Clin Neurosci 1994;6(1):15–22.

54. Langlois JA, Rutland-Brown W, Wald MM. The epidemiology and impact of traumatic brain injury a brief overview. J Head Trauma Rehabil 2006;21(5):375–8.

55. Giza CC, Hovda DA. The new neurometabolic cascade of concussion. Neurosurgery 2014;75:S24–33.

56. Colvin AC, Mullen J, Lovell MR, et al. The role of concussion history and gender in recovery from soccer-related concussion. Am J Sports Med 2009;37(9):1699–704.

57. Lau B, Lovell MR, Collins MW, et al. Neurocognitive and symptom predictors of recovery in high school athletes. Clin J Sport Med 2009;19(3):216–21.

58. Iverson GL, Gaetz M, Lovell MR, et al. Cumulative effects of concussion in amateur athletes. Brain Inj 2004;18(5):433–43.

59. Kutcher JS, Eckner JT. At-risk populations in sports-related concussion. Curr Sports Med Rep 2010;9(1):16–20.

60. Leddy JJ, Baker JG, Kozlowski K, et al. Reliability of a graded exercise test for assessing recovery from concussion. Clin J Sport Med 2011;21:89–94.

61. Leddy JJ, Willer B. Use of graded exercise testing in concussion and return-to-activity management. Curr Sports Med Rep 2013;12(6):370–6.

62. Martland HS. Punch drunk. JAMA 1928;91:1103–7.

63. Martland HS. Intracranial injuries and their sequelae and punch drunk. Ther Intern Dis 1943;3:291–301.

64. Stamm JM, Bourlas AP, Baugh CM, et al. Age of first exposure to football and later-life cognitive impairment in former NFL players. Neurology 2015;84(11):1114–20.

65. Montenigro PH, Corp DT, Stein TD, et al. Chronic traumatic encephalopathy: historical origins and current perspective. Annu Rev Clin Psychol 2015;11:309–30.

66. Mez J, Daneshvar DH. Clinicopathological evaluation of chronic traumatic encephalopathy in players of American Football. JAMA 2017;318(4):360–70.

Conventional Computed Tomography and Magnetic Resonance in Brain Concussion

Juan Nicolas Useche, MD*, Sonia Bermudez, MD

KEYWORDS

- Head injury, closed • Craniocerebral trauma • Brain injuries, traumatic • Contrecoup injury
- Brain concussion • Brain contusion • Multidetector computed tomography
- Magnetic resonance imaging

KEY POINTS

- Brain concussion is responsible for approximately 2.5 million emergency department visits, hospitalizations, and deaths in the United States, accounting for $76.5 billion in health care–related costs in 2010.
- Computed tomography (CT) is the preferred imaging modality for the initial assessment of acute mild traumatic brain injury (mTBI), for repeat evaluation in the presence of neurologic deterioration, and for cautious use in pediatric patients.
- Magnetic resonance (MR) imaging is mostly used in patients with acute mTBI with persistent neurologic findings despite normal initial CT and in the subacute and chronic settings.
- The use of standardized clinical criteria to identify patients who can safely forego unnecessary CT studies has greatly reduced radiation exposure and health care–related costs.
- Advanced MR imaging techniques enable the identification of subtle brain lesions that are not visualized on conventional neuroimaging; however, their routine clinical use is still an area of intense research.

INTRODUCTION

There is a renewed global interest in concussion, not only because the causes and effects are not completely understood but also because of its increased incidence. In 2010, the US Centers for Disease Control and Prevention (CDC) estimated that traumatic brain injuries (TBIs) accounted for approximately 2.5 million emergency department (ED) visits, hospitalizations, and deaths in the United States, either as an isolated injury or in combination with other injuries.[1] The incidence of TBI may be underestimated, especially mild TBI

(mTBI), for 2 main reasons: first, patients may too easily dismiss their symptoms, and, second, they may believe that their work situation could be compromised (eg, military personnel and athletes).[2,3]

TBI can have cognitive, behavioral, emotional, and physical effects on a person's quality of life. Estimates based on data from 2 states in the United States indicated that 3.2 million to 5.3 million people live with a TBI-related disability.[4] In addition, the economic impact is significant; it was estimated to be $76.5 billion in 2010.[5]

Diagnostic and Interventional Imaging Department, El Bosque University, Hospital Universitario Fundacion Santa Fe de Bogota, Calle 119 # 7 – 75, Bogota DC 110111, Colombia
* Corresponding author.
E-mail address: nicolas.useche@radiologiafsfb.org

Neuroimag Clin N Am 28 (2018) 15–29
https://doi.org/10.1016/j.nic.2017.09.006
1052-5149/18/© 2017 Elsevier Inc. All rights reserved.

However, this interest is far from new. Theodore Roosevelt in 1905 was the first president of the United States to convene a White House Conference on concussion in sports, after the American college football season of 1905 left 18 dead and 159 seriously injured.[6] The US government authorized research and public health activities related to TBI with the Traumatic Brain Injury Act of 2008, and, in May 2014, President Barack Obama said, during the White House Conference on Sports Concussions, "Let's keep encouraging our kids to get out there and play sports that they love, and doing it the right way. That's not a job just for parents, but it's a job for all of us."[1,7]

Radiologists and neuroradiologists should also be part of the team, not only through involvement in patient evaluations but also by fostering awareness as parents of young athletes.

CONCUSSION VERSUS MILD TRAUMATIC BRAIN INJURY

TBI has traditionally been classified according to severity. The standardized clinical scale most widely used is the Glasgow Coma Scale (GCS), since its creation in 1974 by Teasdale and Jennet.[8] Classically, an mTBI has been defined as a GCS score of 13 to 15, a moderate TBI is one with a GCS score of 9 to 12, and a severe TBI is indicated by a GCS score of 3 to 8.[9] Some investigators have stated that a GCS score of 13 should not be considered an mTBI, including the American College of Emergency Physicians and the CDC.[10,11] Others require normal noncontrast head computed tomography (NCCT) results or the presence of clinical conditions, such as loss of consciousness (LOC) and amnesia, to make an mTBI diagnosis, thus hampering the collection of comparable epidemiologic and surveillance data.

Some investigators have used the terms concussion and mTBI interchangeably; however, in sports, the last available update in the definition of concussion was at the Fourth International Conference on Concussion in Sport in 2012. Concussion is a complex pathophysiologic process affecting the brain that is caused by biomechanical forces stemming from a direct blow to the head, face, neck, or elsewhere on the body. It results in a spontaneously resolving neurologic impairment of rapid onset, which may evolve over minutes to hours or may present a protracted course, and it may or may not be accompanied by an LOC.[12]

In summary, mTBI is defined as a GCS score between 13 and 15, an LOC of less than 30 minutes, and amnesia of less than 1 day.[1,13] Alternatively, concussion is defined as a brain injury resulting

in a short period of functional neurologic impairment, without conventional neuroimaging evidence of structural damage.[12] This article focuses on conventional neuroimaging techniques and usage in mTBI assessment, considering concussion to be the mildest form of mTBI. In addition, the emphasis is on the acute phase and follow-up of mTBI, because chronic concussion is further discussed elsewhere in this issue.

CONVENTIONAL NEUROIMAGING IN CONCUSSION AND MILD TRAUMATIC BRAIN INJURY

The screening of sport concussions is largely based on the injury mechanism and on the signs and symptoms of neurologic impairment. However, neuroimaging should be used whenever suspicion of an intracerebral or structural lesion exists. These situations include a prolonged disturbance of consciousness, a focal neurologic deficit, or worsening of the initial clinical presentation.[12] Although LOC has been associated with early cognitive findings, its role as a measure of injury severity is controversial. The Zurich Consensus of 2012 determined that an LOC of more than 1 minute should be considered a factor that may modify management.[14,15] Persistent symptoms over more than 10 days are reported in approximately 10% to 15% of patients with concussions and are a reason for further investigation with neuropsychological testing and conventional neuroimaging.[12]

Alternatively, in mTBI, computed tomography (CT) abnormalities, which are also referred to as complicated mTBI, have been detected in up to 5% of patients with a GCS score of 15 and could be as high as 30% in patients with a GCS score of 13.[16–18] According to a meta-analysis by af Geijerstam and Britton,[19] from every 1000 patients arriving with mTBI at a hospital, 1 dies, 9 require surgery, and 80 show pathologic findings on a CT scan. In children with sports-related head trauma who undergo NCCT, 4% had CT abnormalities and 1% were considered clinically significant.[20] Furthermore, patients with abnormal CT findings and a GCS score of 13 or 14 are considered to be at a high risk of undergoing more neurosurgical interventions and having worse outcomes.[21]

Conventional neuroimaging is used as part of the assessment of TBI in the acute, subacute, and chronic settings and during follow-up. The imaging modalities most widely used to assess head trauma CT and magnetic resonance (MR) imaging.

CT is the preferred imaging modality for acute mTBI, for repeat assessment in acute TBI with neurologic deterioration in adults, and for cautious use in pediatric patients with mTBI, according to different clinical guidelines.[3,13,22]

MR imaging is not currently recommended for the primary evaluation of acute TBI. It is used in patients with acute or subacute TBI when initial or follow-up NCCT is normal and there are persistent neurologic findings.[3,23]

Although advanced neuroimaging, including diffusion tensor imaging, functional MR imaging, MR spectroscopy, MR perfusion imaging, PET, single-photon emission CT, and magnetoencephalography, may be more sensitive than conventional imaging in the detection of subtle lesions, there is not sufficient evidence to recommend its routine clinical use in the initial assessment of concussion/mTBI diagnosis and prognostication of individual patients. However, they may provide useful information in patients with no conventional imaging findings.[24]

NEUROIMAGING FOR ACUTE MILD TRAUMATIC BRAIN INJURY
Computed Tomography

The main advantages of CT for initial head trauma evaluation are 2-fold: first, it is a widely available imaging modality, and, second, it permits a rapid evaluation of the patient. It is also compatible with medical and life support devices and does not require screening for the presence of ferromagnetic or metallic materials. It is highly sensitive to the intracranial mass effect, fluid collections, radiopaque foreign bodies, calvarial and skull base fractures, and acute intra-axial or extra-axial hemorrhage, which enables physicians to rule out severe, life-threatening lesions that may require emergent neurosurgical treatment or that may benefit from early aggressive medical therapy or bedside neurologic supervision. The recommended protocol includes 2 sets of images using brain and bone reconstruction algorithms and multiplanar reformatted images (maximum 5-mm thickness) to maximize the sensitivity to detect intracranial hemorrhage (Fig. 1). Wei and colleagues[25] identified 14% more hemorrhages in coronal planes, compared with axial slices, mostly in the floor of the anterior and middle cranial fossae, vertex, corpus callosum, falx, tentorium, and occipital convexity.[25,26] The postprocessing of the image using dedicated bone algorithms and tridimensional renderings facilitated the detection of small fractures in both the calvaria and in the base of the skull (Fig. 2).

The concern for the increased number of CT scans performed in patients with minor head trauma and the risk of ionizing radiation exposure, particularly in young children, has led to an increase in efforts designed to reduce the amount of nonindicated scans.[26] The use of clinical criteria and risk factors to adequately select patients who would benefit from head CT has reduced the number of CT scans performed for mTBI in the acute setting.[27,28] Smits and colleagues[29] estimated that screening patients with the Canadian CT Head Rule (CCHR) could lead to a $120 million reduction in TBI-related health care costs in the United States per year. Furthermore, a recent report that analyzed the contributing factors for CT overuse for minor head injuries in a tertiary hospital found that 37.3% of the requested scans were not indicated according to the CCHR. The

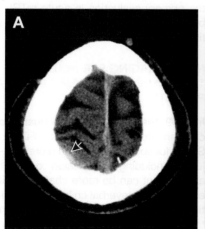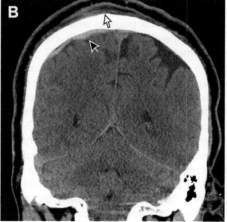

Fig. 1. A 54-year old man with mTBI following a vehicle accident. Head CT. (*A*) Axial and (*B*) coronal images. A small subdural hematoma (*black arrowhead*) is not clearly seen in the axial image. The coronal reformatted image better shows the thickness and extension of the laminar parietal subdural hematoma (*black arrowhead*) and mild adjacent soft tissue edema (*white arrow*).

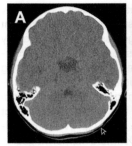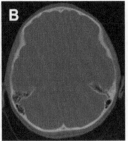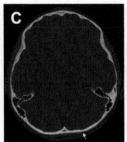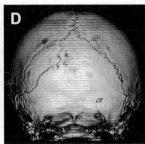

Fig. 2. A 7-year old boy with mTBI after a 1-m fall. Head CT. (*A*) Axial image on soft tissue window. (*B*) Axial image on bone window–soft tissue algorithm. (*C*) Axial image on bone window–bone algorithm. (*D*) Three-dimensional surface shaded display. In *A* there is no evidence of soft tissue abnormalities or of extra-axial collections (*black arrowhead*). In *B* the occipital linear nondisplaced fracture is not visualized as clearly as in *C. D* allows a better evaluation of the extension of the fracture (*white arrow*) that reaches the superior nuchal line, which is at the level of the transverse sinus groove.

most important factors underlying this behavior were physician specialty (ie, neurology overuses CT more than neurosurgery) and injury mechanism (ie, 4-wheel motor vehicle accident and direct blow to the head by an object).[30] The most current issue of the Appropriateness Criteria for Head Trauma from the American College of Radiology (ACR) recommends the use of the CCHR, the New Orleans Criteria (NOC), and the National Emergency X-ray Utilization Study (NEXUS II) to determine which patients with mTBI can safely avoid head NCCT[22,28,31,32] (**Table 1**).

Magnetic Resonance Imaging

MR imaging is currently not recommended for the initial evaluation of acute TBI under many practice guidelines.[13] The main reasons for this strong agreement are that it is not as widely available as CT, it requires longer acquisition times, it has higher sensitivity to patient motion, and it is incompatible with some life support and implanted medical devices. Nevertheless, it has a place in current practice in the evaluation of patients with acute or subacute TBI with persistent neurologic impairment despite normal initial or follow-up NCCT.[3,23]

MR imaging is more sensitive (93%–98%) than CT (18%–56%) in detecting acute and chronic extra-axial traumatic collections and hemorrhagic and nonhemorrhagic contusions, which were more clearly observed in T2-weighted and T2-weighted fluid-attenuation inversion recovery (FLAIR) sequences.[33–35] In addition, all types and stages of intracranial hemorrhage, including subdural and epidural hematomas, subarachnoid hemorrhage (SAH), contusions (particularly those adjacent to bony surfaces), axonal injury, and brainstem lesions, are also better detected with MR.[33–38] Yuh and colleagues,[39] as part of the TRACK/TBI (Transforming Research and Clinical Knowledge in Traumatic Brain Injury)

study, reported MR imaging abnormalities in 28% of patients with normal head CT. Four or more foci of hemorrhagic axonal injury and 1 or more brain contusions on MR imaging are considered independent predictive factors of a poor 3-month outcome, after adjusting for other clinical and head CT findings. Although it is evident that MR imaging is more sensitive than CT for the detection of small brain lesions in mTBI, the clinical utility for clinical decision making in the acute setting is still unclear.[38]

In summary, in the acute setting of mTBI, NCCT is the preferred imaging technique because of a high negative predictive value to exclude the need for neurosurgical intervention. The use of any of the 3 major clinical criteria to select patients with mTBI could safely avoid the use of neuroimaging. Despite the better sensitivity of MR imaging when detecting brain lesions compared with CT, the significance for clinical decision making is unclear. It is currently not recommended for the primary evaluation in acute mTBI, but it may be indicated in patients with persistent neurologic findings.[3,38]

NEUROIMAGING FOR ACUTE MILD TRAUMATIC BRAIN INJURY IN PEDIATRIC PATIENTS

In 2009, there were almost a quarter of a million children admitted and treated at EDs in the United States for sports-related and recreation-related injuries, including concussion or TBI.[40] Clinical assessment can be more challenging in children, especially in preverbal children.[41] Imaging evaluation can also be especially difficult in children less than 18 months old because of incomplete white matter myelination. As in adults, most mTBIs do not require intervention; however, up to 5% of children have abnormalities on imaging and less than 1% require neurosurgical intervention.[42]

Table 1
Clinical rules to identify patients with mild traumatic brain injury who can safely avoid undergoing computed tomography

NOC[¶]	CCHR[†]	NEXUS II[‡]
CT is not required if all of the following are absent		

Headache
Vomiting
Age ≤60 y
Drug or alcohol intoxication
Deficits in short-term memory
Physical evidence of trauma above the clavicles
Seizure
	High-risk factors (for neurologic intervention)
	  GCS score <15 at 2 h after injury
	  Suspected open or depressed skull fracture
	  Any sign of basilar skull fracture[b]
	  Vomiting ≥2 episodes
	  Age ≥65 y
	Medium risk factors (for brain injury on CT)
	  Amnesia before impact >30 min
	  Dangerous mechanism[c]
		Evidence of significant skull fracture
		Scalp hematoma
		Neurologic deficit
		Altered level of alertness
		Abnormal behavior
		Coagulopathy
		Persistent vomiting
		Age ≥65 y

Inclusion Criteria		
Minor head injury[a] Age >3 y Injury within the past 24 h	Blunt trauma to the head resulting in witnessed loss of consciousness, definite amnesia, or witnessed disorientation Initial ED GCS score ≥13 as determined by the treating physician Injury within the past 24 h	Blunt trauma with minor head injury (GCS score 15)
Exclusion Criteria		
Patient preference to decline CT Presence of concurrent injuries that precluded the use of CT No LOC or amnesia for the traumatic event	Age <16 y Minimal head injury (ie, no LOC, amnesia, or disorientation) No clear history of trauma as the primary event (eg, primary seizure or syncope) Obvious penetrating skull injury or obvious depressed fracture Acute focal neurologic deficit Unstable vital signs associated with major trauma Seizure before assessment in the ED Bleeding disorder or usage of oral anticoagulants Return for reassessment of the same head injury Pregnancy	Patients without blunt trauma (including those with penetrating head trauma) Patients undergoing head CT imaging for other reasons

[a] LOC in patients with normal findings on a brief neurologic examination (normal cranial nerves and normal strength and sensation in the arms and legs) and a GCS score of 15, as determined by a physician on the patient's arrival at the ED.
[b] Hemotympanum, racoon eyes, cerebrospinal fluid otorrhea/rhinorrhea, Battle sign.
[c] Pedestrian struck by motor vehicle, occupant ejected from motor vehicle, fall from height greater than 1 m (3 feet) or 5 stairs.
Data from Refs.[28,31,32]

The purpose of imaging is to exclude the presence of lesions that require neurosurgical interventions or that may benefit from early medical treatment. CT evaluation has been the reference standard for the evaluation of acute brain injury in children.[43] From 1995 to 2003, the use of CT increased from 13% to 22%, raising concern about ionizing radiation exposure.[44] The estimated risk of induced lethal malignancy in children is 1 in 1000 to 1 in 5000 per cranial CT.[26] Thus, efforts to reduce radiation doses have been pursued; for example, Kahn and colleagues[45] reported 23% of applied doses without loss of image quality in whole-body CT protocols in patients with trauma using an adaptive statistical iterative reconstruction. The Society of Pediatric Radiology and the ACR (Image Gently) have developed dedicated pediatric CT protocols that are tailored by patient size to avoid unnecessarily high radiation doses.[46]

Other efforts focused on reducing the number of CT scans for evaluating children with acute head trauma have been performed. As in adults, clinical decision rules have been used to identify children with clinically significant TBI presenting to the ED after a minor head trauma. The

Children's Head Injury Algorithm for the Prediction of Important Clinical Events (CHALICE) rule,[47] the Canadian Assessment of Tomography for Childhood Head injury (CATCH) rule,[48] and the Pediatric Emergency Care Applied Research Network (PECARN) rule[42] are the most commonly used. A prospective study from Easter and colleagues[49] compared the diagnostic accuracy of clinical decision rules and physician judgment in the identification of clinically important traumatic brain injuries (GCS scores 13–15) in children (<18 years old) with mTBI presenting to the ED within 24 hours of injury by comparing the ability of the CHALICE, CATCH, and PECARN rules and 2 measures of physician judgment (CT ordering practice and estimated a <1% risk of TBI). Clinically important brain injuries were defined by death, the need for neurosurgical intervention, intubation greater than 24 hours, or hospital admission greater than 2 nights for TBI. The investigators identified sensitivities of 100% for clinically important TBI with PECARN and physician practice, whereas PECARN was barely more specific. CHALICE was the most specific, but it had a sensitivity of 84%.[49] Later, Nishijima and colleagues[50] conducted a cost-effectiveness analysis comparing PECARN rules with usual care for selective CT use and found that application of the PECARN rules in children with mTBI leads to better outcomes and more cost-effective care, reducing the number of CT scans performed and resulting in fewer radiation-induced cancers. The PECARN study was performed to identify children at a very low risk of clinically important TBI (ciTBI) for whom CT might be unnecessary. Patients were enrolled (42,412) and divided into 2 groups: younger than 2 years and from 2 to 18 years. Both groups had GCS scores of 14 to 15. The investigators found that 0.9% had ciTBI and that 0.1% underwent neurosurgery. Using the prediction rules to select children (Table 2), approximately 25% of the CT scans in those younger than 2 years and 20% in those aged 2 years and older could be avoided. Patients with GCS score less than 15 or with palpable or basilar skull fractures had an approximately 4.4% risk of ciTBI, whereas patients with any isolated clinical finding, as stated in the second part of Table 2, had a 0.9% risk of ciTBI. In this subgroup of patients, observation without CT might be appropriate, considering clinician experience, worsening of symptoms or signs after clinical observation, and parental preferences.[42]

The last update of the Appropriateness Criteria for Head Trauma in children from the ACR considered the use of NCCT in patients older than

Table 2
The Pediatric Emergency Care Applied Research Network prediction rules for identifying children at very low risk of clinically important traumatic brain injury for whom computed tomography can routinely be avoided

Children Aged <2 y	Children Aged ≥2 y
CT recommended in the presence of any of these findings (ciTBI risk is approximately 4.4%)	
GCS = 14 or other signs of altered mental status	GCS = 14 or other signs of altered mental status
Palpable skull fracture	Signs of basilar skull fracture
CT vs observation depending on the presence of these findings and certain clinical factors[a] (ciTBI risk is 0.9%)	
Scalp hematoma, except frontal	History of LOC
History of LOC ≥5 s	History of vomiting
Severe injury mechanism[b]	Severe mechanism of injury[b]
Not acting normally according to parents	Severe headache
NPV = 100%	NPV = 99.95%
Sensitivity = 100%	Sensitivity = 96.8%

Abbreviation: NPV, negative predictive value.
[a] Clinical factors include physician experience, multiple versus isolated findings, worsening symptoms or signs after ED observation, age less than 3 months, parental preference.
[b] Severe injury mechanisms include motor vehicle crash with patient ejection, death of another passenger, or rollover; pedestrian or bicyclist without helmet struck by a motorized vehicle; falls of more than 1.5 m (5 feet) for children aged 2 years and older and more than 0.9 m (3 feet) for those younger than 2 years; or head struck by a high-impact object.
Data from Kuppermann N, Holmes JF, Dayan PS, et al. Identification of children at very low risk of clinically-important brain injuries after head trauma: a prospective cohort study. Lancet 2009;374(9696):1160–70.

2 years with minor head injury (ie, GCS scores of 14–15), without neurologic signs or high-risk factors (ie, altered mental status [AMS] or clinical evidence of basilar skull fracture), and in patients younger than 2 years with minor head injury to be usually not appropriate without neurologic signs or high-risk factors. In contrast, in patients with minor head trauma but with any of the same high-risk factors, NCCT is considered usually appropriate. In pediatric patients, despite radiation concerns, CT remains the primary modality for evaluating suspected acute intracranial injury in most instances. Although MR has equal or higher sensitivity for the detection of intracranial hemorrhage and traumatic parenchymal lesions, reports suggest that they are often not clinically significant. In a prospective study evaluating 13,543 children with mTBI, no patients with initial negative NCCT required neurosurgical intervention.[51]

NEUROIMAGING FOR FOLLOW-UP IN MILD TRAUMATIC BRAIN INJURY

The decision to obtain follow-up images in TBI depends mostly on whether there is neurologic deterioration. A systematic review of the literature performed by Stippler and colleagues[52] found that routine follow-up head CT did not predict the need for neurosurgical intervention ($P = .10$), whereas head CT performed for decline status did ($P = .00046$). Patients receiving anticoagulation therapy, older than 65 years, or with subfrontal or temporal intraparenchymal contusion also benefitted from follow-up NCCT.[53,54] However, recent evidence suggested that patients on anticoagulation therapy with mTBI and a GCS score of 15 had a similar risk to that of nonanticoagulated patients; it may be reasonable to forego a repeat head CT scan while remaining under appropriate observation.[55]

In a retrospective review of 321 patients in a level 1 trauma center over a 2-year period, patients with mTBI did not require surgical intervention. Even patients with initial abnormal CT (ie, convexity SAH, small convexity contusion, intraparenchymal hematoma of <10 mL, and small subdural hematomas) and no clinical deterioration required intensive care unit (ICU) admission or repeat imaging.[54] The meta-analysis of Reljic and colleagues,[56] which evaluated 10,501 patients, found that, in the subgroup of patients with mTBI, repeating an NCCT scan resulted in a change in management in less than 4% of patients in prospective and retrospective studies. Thus, follow-up NCCT in patients with mTBI and no clinical deterioration is not

recommended.[3] MR is recommended in patients with ongoing neurologic or progressive neurologic symptoms unexplained by CT. Contrast-enhanced brain MR is recommended if infection is suspected.[22]

In pediatric patients, follow-up imaging is less supported than in adults. According to Durham and colleagues,[57] in 268 children with TBI, follow-up CT was recommended for patients with epidural, subdural, and parenchymal hematomas, as well as brain edema; in patients with SAH, IVH, diffuse axonal injury (DAI), and isolated skull fractures without clinical deterioration, the follow-up CT scan was less likely to change clinical management. A recent study found that adverse events after nonoperative mTBI in pediatric patients were rare and that routine follow-up neuroimaging did not influence delayed operative intervention.[58] To summarize, the most recent ACR recommendations for acute and follow-up conventional imaging in concussion/mTBI are shown in **Table 3**.

CONVENTIONAL IMAGING FINDINGS: MECHANISM OF INJURY AND MOST COMMON LESIONS

Concussion is a type of mTBI that most frequently presents among young people and is usually related to sport trauma (eg, football, ice hockey, boxing, wrestling, and car racing). Brain injury occurs secondary to translational and rotational acceleration vectors causing either coup or contrecoup injury. More specifically, the intracranial pressure gradient created by the linear accelerating/deaccelerating forces are the cause of parenchymal contusions, whereas the rotational vectors are responsible for most axonal shear injury.[59] However, evidence suggests that rotational acceleration has a more important role in the biomechanics of concussion than translational acceleration alone, which has led to the development of better and safer protection gear and helmets.[60,61] Moreover, advances in the understanding of mechanically induced neuronal cytoskeletal deformability have elucidated cellular and molecular mechanisms that underpin white matter loss and subsequent progressive cognitive decline as a late complication of TBI. In this respect, dedicated MR imaging techniques have proved to be the imaging modality of choice, thus becoming an area of intense research focus, as discussed further elsewhere in this issue.[38] Nevertheless, conventional MR imaging is important in specific situations in trauma assessment and in the evaluation of axonal injury.[62]

Table 3
Conventional neuroimaging in acute and follow-up concussion/mild traumatic brain injury based on the American College of Radiology Appropriateness Criteria recommendations

Variant	NCCT	MR Imaging
Adult		
Minor or mild acute closed head injury (GCS score ≥13), imaging not indicated by NOC or CCHR or NEXUS II clinical criteria	2	1
Minor or mild acute closed head injury (GCS score ≥13), imaging indicated by NOC or CCHR or NEXUS II clinical criteria	9	5
Short-term follow-up imaging of acute TBI (no neurologic deterioration)[a]	5	2
Short-term follow-up imaging of acute TBI (neurologic deterioration, delayed recovery, or persistent unexplained deficits)	9	8
Pediatric[†]		
Minor head injury (GCS score >13) at ≥2 y of age without neurologic signs or high-risk factors.[b] Excluding nonaccidental trauma	3	2
Minor head injury (GCS score >13) at <2 y of age, no neurologic signs or high-risk factors.[b] Excluding nonaccidental trauma	3	3
Minor head trauma with high-risk factors.[b] Excluding nonaccidental trauma	9	7

Rating scale: 1, 2, and 3 = usually not appropriate; 4, 5, and 6 = may be appropriate; 7, 8, and 9 = usually appropriate.
  [a] Unless a patient has subfrontal or temporal intraparenchymal contusions, is anticoagulated, is >65 years of age, or has an intracranial hemorrhage with a volume of greater than 10 mL.
  [b] AMS, clinical evidence of basilar skull fracture.
  Data from Shetty VS, Reis MN, Aulino JM, et al. ACR appropriateness criteria head trauma. J Am Coll Radiol 2016;13(6):668–79; and Ryan ME, Palasis S, Saigal G, et al. ACR appropriateness criteria head trauma–child. J Am Coll Radiol 2014;11(10):939–47.

IMAGING FINDINGS IN CONCUSSION AND TRAUMATIC BRAIN INJURY

The National Institute of Neurological Disorders and Stroke (NINDS) has developed TBI common data elements to streamline research through the use of universal data standards.[63] In keeping with this guideline, this article uses the same definitions and describes the lesions most frequently encountered in concussion and mTBI.

Skull Fractures

Linear and branched fracture lines are more frequent in minor trauma than displaced fractures, and they are better appreciated using dedicated bone algorithms, multiplanar reformatted images, and tridimensional renderings. Companion signs to increase awareness of skull fractures often include subgaleal hematomas, adjacent pneumocephalus, or extra-axial hemorrhagic collections. In children, multiplanar reformatted images help to distinguish them from sutures. Infants are more susceptible to calvarial fracture than older children because the fracture threshold for an infant is approximately 10% that of an older child or adult. The prevalence of fractures has been reported to be 11% in children younger than 2 years, compared with a 2% prevalence in all children.[26]

Isolated nondepressed skull fractures typically do not need specific therapy or hospital admission; however, if they are next to vascular structures, they may be associated with vascular injury (see **Fig. 2**).

Extra-Axial Collections

When the exact location cannot be determined, the recommended term is extra-axial collections. In the mTBI setting, epidural and subdural hematomas are usually small and linear (**Fig. 3**), whereas SAH is commonly found in the convexities of the brain (**Fig. 4**). Most of these lesions are treated conservatively; however, epidural hematomas could progress and should be considered in a different subgroup when follow-up imaging is performed.[64] Identification of such intracranial hemorrhagic lesions on the admission CT scan is of the utmost important. Although it may not acutely change clinical management, intracranial abnormalities have been correlated with acute and long-term neuropsychiatric deficits following mTBI.[54,65]

Parenchymal Contusions

Small intraparenchymal hemorrhagic contusions are a common finding in complicated mTBI (**Fig. 5**) and are frequently located near the site of

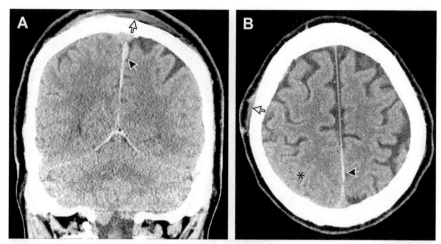

Fig. 3. A 54-year old man with mTBI following a vehicle accident. Head CT. (*A*) Coronal and (*B*) axial images show a linear high density with mild thickening of the falx caused by a small subdural hematoma (*black arrowhead*). Right parietal sulci effacement consistent with mild brain parenchymal edema (*asterisk*) without evidence of focal contusion. Right parietal soft tissue swelling (*white arrow*).

coup or contrecoup injury, in the anterior temporal and frontal poles, and in the fronto-orbital gyri. Although small contusions may not be clinically significant, there are reports of lesion progression in up to 53% of patients with subfrontal or temporal intraparenchymal contusions that required changes in acute management, such as ICU admission or repeat imaging.[54]

Axonal Injury

Mechanical strain caused by rotational acceleration/deceleration forces underlies the pathophysiology of the scattered, small, white matter lesions found in mTBI. DAI refers to the widespread presence of more than 3 foci of white matter signal abnormality, whereas traumatic axonal injury (TAI) refers to the presence of up to 3 similar lesions in a more confined distribution. This type of lesion primarily affects the parasagittal white matter, most commonly the subcortical frontal and periventricular temporal, internal capsule, posterior aspect of the corpus callosum and fornix, and dorsolateral and rostral brainstem.[63] Axonal injury appears as hypodense or hyperdense white matter foci on CT scans (**Fig. 6**). Several MR techniques, including FLAIR, diffusion-weighted imaging (DWI), gradient-echo

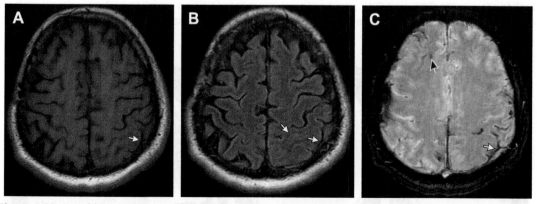

Fig. 4. A 39-year old man with memory loss following an mTBI. Brain MR imaging (*A*) T1-weighted spin echo image. (*B*) T2-weighted FLAIR image. (*C*) Susceptibility-weighted imaging (SWI). Left parietal sulci with no abnormality in T1-weighted, an intermediate signal in T2-weighted FLAIR, and low signal in SWI images (*white arrows*) consistent with a minimal convexity SAH, better evaluated in *C*. A right subcortical frontal white matter punctate focus of low signal (*black arrowhead*) consistent with TAI. This finding was not detectable in the other MR imaging.

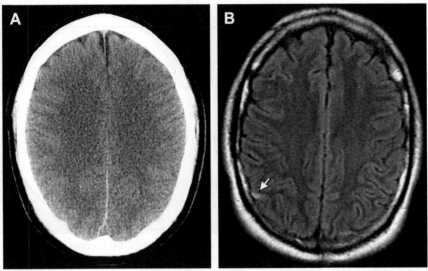

Fig. 5. A 36-year old man with mTBI, LOC, and diplopia following a car crash. (*A*) Head CT, axial projection on brain window. (*B*) MR imaging T2-weighted FLAIR axial image. The small right parietal contusion (*white arrow*) clearly seen on MR imaging was not visible on the CT image.

(GRE) sequences, and susceptibility-weighted imaging (SWI), are especially helpful in identifying hemorrhagic and nonhemorrhagic axonal injuries and should be included in the conventional imaging protocols in mTBI (**Fig. 7**).[66] Although their utility for clinical decision making in the acute setting is still unclear, some investigators have found that the number of TAI lesions in DWI and the volume of lesions in FLAIR in the corpus callosum, brain stem, and thalamus were independent prognostic factors in TBI, emphasizing the importance of the use of conventional MR sequences in TBI.[38,67] In sports concussion, they can also influence the clinical decision about return to play.[68] T2* GRE and SWI sequences are of paramount importance for evaluating DAI.

SWI uses magnitude and phase information, and it is more sensitive than T2* GRE sequences for depicting size, number, and volume of DAI lesions.[69] Magnet field strength is also important; 7-T magnets are superior to both 3-T and 1.5-T magnets when visualizing hemorrhagic DAI lesions.[70,71] SWI may be useful to differentiate DAI and fat embolism in patients with mTBI and unexplained neurologic deficits on CT. Most commonly, focal SWI lesions in DAI are bigger and mostly involve white matter, whereas fat embolism lesions appear more extensive, punctate, and smaller, and involve basal ganglia and cerebellum more frequently than DAI (**Fig. 8**).[72] The most common conventional neuroimaging findings are summarized in **Box 1**.

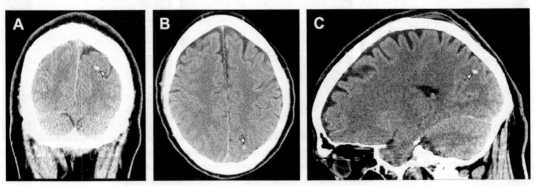

Fig. 6. A 54-year old man with mTBI following a vehicle accident. Head CT. (*A*) Coronal, (*B*) axial, and (*C*) sagittal images. Images show a left parietal subcortical hyperdense focus (*white arrows*) consistent with a hemorrhagic TAI. Mild parietal soft tissue edema is also seen.

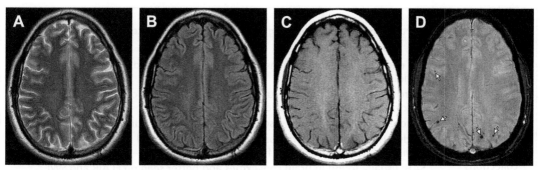

Fig. 7. Brain MR imaging of a 33-year old man with complaints of lack of concentration following a motor vehicle accident. (*A*) T2-weighted axial, (*B*) T2-weighted FLAIR axial, (*C*) T1-weighted axial, and (*D*) SWI axial images. Small foci of signal abnormality (*white arrows*) consistent with hemosiderin deposition as a DAI sequela, visualized in SWI but not in the other MR sequences.

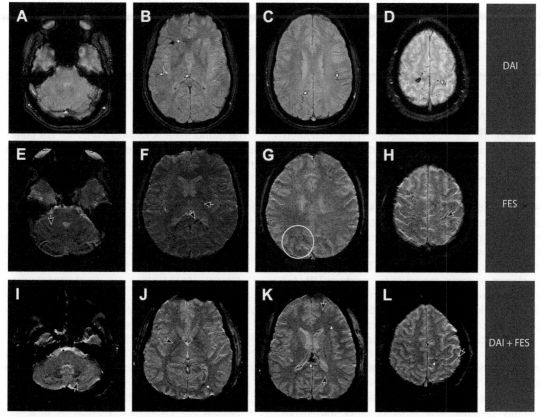

Fig. 8. (*A–D*) SWI axial images of a patient after a motor race accident. (*E–H*) SWI axial images after a sport trauma with a GCS score of 15 and an associated tibia fracture. (*I–L*) SWI axial images of a patient after a severe head injury caused by a motor vehicle accident. The first 4 images show small rounded foci of susceptibility artifact involving the subcortical white matter without cerebellar involvement, consistent with grade I DAI (*white arrows*). The next 4 images show punctate extensive foci with less susceptibility artifact involving the peripheral gray matter, the white matter of the centrum semiovale (*circle*), the corpus callosum, the basal ganglia, and the gray and white matter of the cerebellum (*black arrows*), consistent with fat embolism. The last 4 images show the same characteristic findings just described, consistent with coexistent DAI (*white arrows*) and fat embolism (*black arrows*) in the same patient.

Box 1
Summary of most important information regarding lesions associated with concussion/mild traumatic brain injury

Skull fractures	Use dedicated bone algorithms, multiplanar reformatted images, and tridimensional renderings
	Search for companion signs: subgaleal hematomas, adjacent pneumocephalus, extra-axial hemorrhagic collections
	Children <2 y old are more susceptible to calvarial fractures than older patients
Extra-axial hemorrhagic collections	Epidural and subdural hematomas: frequently small and linear, intermediate window helps differentiate from adjacent bone
	SAH: usually found in brain convexities and better seen on FLAIR and SWI
Parenchymal contusions	Frequently located near the site of coup and contrecoup injury, in the anterior temporal and frontal poles, and in the fronto-orbital gyri
	About half of subfrontal and temporal contusions may require ICU admission or repeated imaging
Axonal injury	Found in the parasagittal, subcortical frontal, and periventricular temporal white matter; internal capsule; posterior aspect of corpus callosum; fornix; and dorsolateral and rostral brainstem
	TAI: $\leq$3 foci of white matter signal abnormality in a defined brain region
	DAI: >3 foci of white matter signal abnormality in a widespread distribution
	SWI sequence and higher field strength magnets improve its rates of detection
	SWI could differentiate it from fat embolism lesions, which are more punctate and have a more extensive distribution, often involving the basal ganglia and cerebellum

---

SUMMARY

There is still controversy between the definition of concussion and mTBI. The screening of sport brain concussion is largely based on injury mechanism and on signs and symptoms of neurologic impairment. However, neuroimaging should be used whenever suspicion of an intracranial structural lesion exists. Conventional neuroimaging is still the mainstay in the assessment of the acute, follow-up, and chronic settings of concussion and mTBI. CT is the preferred imaging modality for acute mTBI, for repeat assessment in acute mTBI with neurologic deterioration, and for cautious use in pediatric patients with mTBI. MR imaging is mostly used in patients with acute, subacute, or chronic mTBI when initial or follow-up NCCT scans are normal and there are persistent neurologic findings.

Several clinical rules have been developed to identify pediatric and adult patients with mTBI who can safely forego an NCCT scan. Knowledge of the mechanism of injury and most common findings in conventional CT and MR are pivotal for image interpretation in mTBI. The role of advanced imaging techniques in the assessment of mTBI and concussion, which remains an area of intense research, is discussed in detail in other articles of this issue.

ACKNOWLEDGMENTS

The authors thank Nicolas Yanez for his contributions in reviewing and editing the article, tables, and figures.

REFERENCES

1. US Centers for Disease Control and Prevention. Report to Congress on Traumatic Brain Injury in the United States: epidemiology and rehabilitation. National Center for Injury Prevention and Control. 2015;Division of Unintentional Injury Prevention.

2. Ilie G, Boak A, Adlaf EM, et al. Prevalence and correlates of traumatic brain injuries among adolescents. JAMA 2013;309(24):2550–2.

3. Wintermark M, Sanelli PC, Anzai Y, et al. Imaging evidence and recommendations for traumatic brain injury: conventional neuroimaging techniques. J Am Coll Radiol 2015;12(2):e1–14.

4. Selassie AW, Zaloshnja E, Langlois JA, et al. Incidence of long-term disability following traumatic brain injury hospitalization, United States, 2003. J Head Trauma Rehabil 2008;23(2):123–31.

5. Centers for Disease Control and Prevention (CDC). Homicide rates among persons aged 10–24 years — United States, 1981–2010 [Internet]. MMWR Morb Mortal Wkly Rep 2013; 62(27):545–8.

6. Stone JL, Patel V, Bailes JE. The history of neurosurgical treatment of sports concussion. Neurosurgery 2014;75(Suppl 4):S3–23.

7. The White House Office of the Press Secretary. Remarks by the President at the Healthy Kids and Safe Sports concussion summit [Internet]. The White House Office of the Press Secretary; 2014.

8. Teasdale G, Jennett B. Assessment of coma and impaired consciousness. A practical scale. Lancet 1974;2(7872):81–4.

9. Cushman JG, Agarwal N, Fabian TC, et al. Practice management guidelines for the management of mild traumatic brain injury: the EAST Practice Management Guidelines Work Group. J Trauma 2001; 51(5):1016–26.

10. Stein SC. Minor head injury: 13 is an unlucky number. J Trauma 2001;50(4):759–60.

11. Jagoda AS, Bazarian JJ, Bruns JJ Jr, et al. Clinical policy: neuroimaging and decisionmaking in adult mild traumatic brain injury in the acute setting. Ann Emerg Med 2008;52(6):714–48.

12. McCrory P, Meeuwisse WH, Aubry M, et al. Consensus statement on concussion in sport: the 4th International Conference on Concussion in Sport held in Zurich, November 2012. Br J Sports Med 2013;47(5):250–8.

13. Tavender EJ, Bosch M, Green S, et al. Quality and consistency of guidelines for the management of mild traumatic brain injury in the emergency department. Acad Emerg Med 2011;18(8):880–9.

14. Lovell MR, Iverson GL, Collins MW, et al. Does loss of consciousness predict neuropsychological decrements after concussion? Clin J Sport Med 1999; 9(4);193–8.

15. McCrory P, Meeuwisse W, Johnston K, et al. Consensus statement on concussion in sport: the 3rd International Conference on Concussion in Sport held in Zurich, November 2008. Br J Sports Med 2009;43(Suppl 1):i76–90.

16. Rosenbaum SB, Lipton ML. Embracing chaos: the scope and importance of clinical and pathological heterogeneity in mTBI. Brain Imaging Behav 2012; 6(2):255–82.

17. Zafonte R, Eisenberg H. The horizon of neuroimaging for mild TBI. Brain Imaging Behav 2012;6(2): 355–6.

18. Borg J, Holm L, Cassidy JD, et al. Diagnostic procedures in mild traumatic brain injury: results of the WHO Collaborating Centre Task Force on Mild Traumatic Brain Injury. J Rehabil Med 2004;(43 Suppl):61–75.

19. af Geijerstam JL, Britton M. Mild head injury - mortality and complication rate: meta-analysis of findings in a systematic literature review. Acta Neurochir (Wien) 2003;145(10):843–50 [discussion: 850].

20. Glass T, Ruddy RM, Alpern ER, et al. Traumatic brain injuries and computed tomography use in pediatric sports participants. Am J Emerg Med 2015;33(10): 1458–64.

21. Hsiang JN, Yeung T, Yu AL, et al. High-risk mild head injury. J Neurosurg 1997;87(2):234–8.

22. Shetty VS, Reis MN, Aulino JM, et al. ACR appropriateness criteria head trauma. J Am Coll Radiol 2016; 13(6):668–79.

23. Kara A, Celik SE, Dalbayrak S, et al. Magnetic resonance imaging finding in severe head injury patients with normal computerized tomography. Turk Neurosurg 2008;18(1):1–9.

24. Wintermark M, Sanelli PC, Anzai Y, et al, American College of Radiology Head Injury Institute. Imaging evidence and recommendations for traumatic brain injury: advanced neuro- and neurovascular imaging techniques. AJNR Am J Neuroradiol 2015;36(2):E1–11.

25. Wei SC, Ulmer S, Lev MH, et al. Value of coronal reformations in the CT evaluation of acute head trauma. AJNR Am J Neuroradiol 2010;31(2):334–9.

26. Ryan ME, Palasis S, Saigal G, et al. ACR appropriateness criteria head trauma–child. J Am Coll Radiol 2014;11(10):939–47.

27. Miller EC, Holmes JF, Derlet RW. Utilizing clinical factors to reduce head CT scan ordering for minor head trauma patients. J Emerg Med 1997;15(4): 453–7.

28. Stiell IG, Wells GA, Vandemheen K, et al. The Canadian CT Head Rule for patients with minor head injury. Lancet 2001;357(9266):1391–6.

29. Smits M, Dippel DW, Nederkoorn PJ, et al. Minor head injury: CT-based strategies for management– a cost-effectiveness analysis. Radiology 2010; 254(2):532–40.

30. Klang E, Beytelman A, Greenberg D, et al. Overuse of head CT examinations for the investigation of minor head trauma: analysis of contributing factors. J Am Coll Radiol 2017;14(2):171–6.

31. Haydel MJ, Preston CA, Mills TJ, et al. Indications for computed tomography in patients with minor head injury. N Engl J Med 2000;343(2):100–5.

32. Mower WR, Hoffman JR, Herbert M, et al. Developing a decision instrument to guide computed tomographic imaging of blunt head injury patients. J Trauma 2005;59(4):954–9.

33. Gentry LR, Godersky JC, Thompson B, et al. Prospective comparative study of intermediate-field MR and CT in the evaluation of closed head trauma. AJR Am J Roentgenol 1988;150(3):673–82.

34. Kelly AB, Zimmerman RD, Snow RB, et al. Head trauma: comparison of MR and CT–experience in 100 patients. AJNR Am J Neuroradiol 1988;9(4): 699–708.

35. Hesselink JR, Dowd CF, Healy ME, et al. MR imaging of brain contusions: a comparative study with CT. AJR Am J Roentgenol 1988;150(5): 1133–42.

36. Haacke EM, Mittal S, Wu Z, et al. Susceptibility-weighted imaging: technical aspects and clinical applications, part 1. AJNR Am J Neuroradiol 2009; 30(1):19–30.

37. Mittal S, Wu Z, Neelavalli J, et al. Susceptibility-weighted imaging: technical aspects and clinical applications, part 2. AJNR Am J Neuroradiol 2009; 30(2):232–52.

38. Provenzale JM. Imaging of traumatic brain injury: a review of the recent medical literature. AJR Am J Roentgenol 2010;194(1):16–9.

39. Yuh EL, Mukherjee P, Lingsma HF, et al. Magnetic resonance imaging improves 3-month outcome prediction in mild traumatic brain injury. Ann Neurol 2013;73(2):224–35.

40. Centers for Disease Control and Prevention. Nonfatal traumatic brain injuries related to sports and recreation activities among persons aged ≤19 years — United States, 2001–2009. MMWR Morb Mortal Wkly Rep 2011;60(39):1337–42.

41. Schnadower D, Vazquez H, Lee J, et al. Controversies in the evaluation and management of minor blunt head trauma in children. Curr Opin Pediatr 2007;19(3):258–64.

42. Kuppermann N, Holmes JF, Dayan PS, et al. Identification of children at very low risk of clinically-important brain injuries after head trauma: a prospective cohort study. Lancet 2009;374(9696): 1160–70.

43. Toyama Y, Kobayashi T, Nishiyama Y, et al. CT for acute stage of closed head injury. Radiat Med 2005;23(5):309–16.

44. Blackwell CD, Gorelick M, Holmes JF, et al. Pediatric head trauma: changes in use of computed tomography in emergency departments in the United States over time. Ann Emerg Med 2007;49(3):320–4.

45. Kahn J, Grupp U, Kaul D, et al. Computed tomography in trauma patients using iterative reconstruction: reducing radiation exposure without loss of image quality. Acta Radiol 2016;57(3):362–9.

46. Image Gently. The alliance for radiation safety in pediatric imaging. Image gently and CT scans. 2014.

47. Dunning J, Daly JP, Lomas JP, et al. Derivation of the children's head injury algorithm for the prediction of important clinical events decision rule for head injury in children. Arch Dis Child 2006;91(11):885–91.

48. Osmond MH, Klassen TP, Wells GA, et al. CATCH: a clinical decision rule for the use of computed tomography in children with minor head injury. CMAJ 2010; 182(4):341–8.

49. Easter JS, Bakes K, Dhaliwal J, et al. Comparison of PECARN, CATCH, and CHALICE rules for children with minor head injury: a prospective cohort study. Ann Emerg Med 2014;64(2):145–52, 152.e1-5.

50. Nishijima DK, Yang Z, Urbich M, et al. Cost-effectiveness of the PECARN rules in children with minor head trauma. Ann Emerg Med 2015;65(1):72–80.e6.

51. Holmes JF, Borgialli DA, Nadel FM, et al. Do children with blunt head trauma and normal cranial computed tomography scan results require hospitalization for neurologic observation? Ann Emerg Med 2011;58(4):315–22.

52. Stippler M, Smith C, McLean AR, et al. Utility of routine follow-up head CT scanning after mild traumatic brain injury: a systematic review of the literature. Emerg Med J 2012;29(7):528–32.

53. Brown CV, Zada G, Salim A, et al. Indications for routine repeat head computed tomography (CT) stratified by severity of traumatic brain injury. J Trauma 2007;62(6):1339–44 [discussion: 1344–5].

54. Washington CW, Grubb RL Jr. Are routine repeat imaging and intensive care unit admission necessary in mild traumatic brain injury? J Neurosurg 2012; 116(3):549–57.

55. Uccella L, Zoia C, Perlasca F, et al. Mild traumatic brain injury in patients on long-term anticoagulation therapy: do they really need repeated head CT scan? World Neurosurg 2016;93:100–3.

56. Reljic T, Mahony H, Djulbegovic B, et al. Value of repeat head computed tomography after traumatic brain injury: systematic review and meta-analysis. J Neurotrauma 2014;31(1):78–98.

57. Durham SR, Liu KC, Selden NR. Utility of serial computed tomography imaging in pediatric patients with head trauma. J Neurosurg 2006;105(5 Suppl): 365–9.

58. Chern JJ, Sarda S, Howard BM, et al. Utility of surveillance imaging after minor blunt head trauma. J Neurosurg Pediatr 2014;14(3):306–10.

59. Rowson S, Bland ML, Campolettano ET, et al. Biomechanical perspectives on concussion in sport. Sports Med Arthrosc 2016;24(3):100–7.

60. Viano DC, Casson IR, Pellman EJ. Concussion in professional football: biomechanics of the struck player–part 14. Neurosurgery 2007;61(2):313–27 [discussion: 327–8].

61. Hoshizaki TB, Post A, Oeur RA, et al. Current and future concepts in helmet and sports injury prevention. Neurosurgery 2014;75(Suppl 4): S136–48.

62. Chiara Ricciardi M, Bokkers RP, Butman JA, et al. Trauma-specific brain abnormalities in suspected mild traumatic brain injury patients identified in the first 48 hours after injury: a blinded magnetic resonance imaging comparative study including suspected acute minor stroke patients. J Neurotrauma 2017;34(1):23–30.

63. Haacke EM, Duhaime AC, Gean AD, et al. Common data elements in radiologic imaging of traumatic brain injury. J Magn Reson Imaging 2010;32(3): 516–43.

64. Basamh M, Robert A, Lamoureux J, et al. Epidural hematoma treated conservatively: when to expect the worst. Can J Neurol Sci 2016;43(1):74–81.

65. Sadowski-Cron C, Schneider J, Senn P, et al. Patients with mild traumatic brain injury: immediate and long-term outcome compared to intracranial injuries on CT scan. Brain Inj 2006; 20(11):1131–7.

66. Rose SC, Schaffer CE, Young JA, et al. Utilization of conventional neuroimaging following youth concussion. Brain Inj 2017;31:1–7.

67. Moen KG, Brezova V, Skandsen T, et al. Traumatic axonal injury: the prognostic value of lesion load in corpus callosum, brain stem, and thalamus in different magnetic resonance imaging sequences. J Neurotrauma 2014;31(17):1486–96.

68. Ellis MJ, Leiter J, Hall T, et al. Neuroimaging findings in pediatric sports-related concussion. J Neurosurg Pediatr 2015;16(3):241–7.

69. Tong KA, Ashwal S, Holshouser BA, et al. Diffuse axonal injury in children: clinical correlation with hemorrhagic lesions. Ann Neurol 2004;56(1): 36–50.

70. Scheid R, Ott DV, Roth H, et al. Comparative magnetic resonance imaging at 1.5 and 3 Tesla for the evaluation of traumatic microbleeds. J Neurotrauma 2007;24(12):1811–6.

71. Moenninghoff C, Kraff O, Maderwald S, et al. Diffuse axonal injury at ultra-high field MRI. PLoS One 2015; 10(3):e0122329.

72. Bodanapally UK, Shanmuganathan K, Saksobhavivat N, et al. MR imaging and differentiation of cerebral fat embolism syndrome from diffuse axonal injury: application of diffusion tensor imaging. Neuroradiology 2013;55(6):771–8.

Multimodal Advanced Imaging for Concussion

Khader M. Hasan, PhD[a],*, Zafer Keser, MD[b],
Paul E. Schulz, MD[b], Elisabeth A. Wilde, PhD[c,d,e]

KEYWORDS

- Concussion • Multimodal imaging • Traumatic brain injury (TBI) • Quantitative MR imaging
- Cortical thickness • Diffusion tensor imaging (DTI) • Kurtosis • Intravoxel incoherent motion (IVIM)

KEY POINTS

- The potential utility of multimodal imaging is not limited to diagnosis: It can also be beneficial in predicting the clinical course of concussion, monitoring recovery, and assessing the efficacy of existing and developing therapies.
- The pathologic hallmarks of primary and secondary injuries may not be directly measured by conventional clinical protocols, which may contribute to our current problems predicting clinical outcomes. Advanced imaging models of the underlying biochemical mechanisms may be needed.
- The authors emphasize the value of using multimodal and multidimensional quantitative MR imaging methods to improve pathologic specificity and potential in predicting clinical outcomes.

INTRODUCTION

Overall, the yearly worldwide incidence of traumatic brain injury (TBI) is estimated to be around 10 million (Murray 1996). Motor vehicle accidents (MVA), sporting events, falls, violence, war, and other unintentional injuries have been postulated as the most common causes of TBI in the literature. The highest rates of TBI due to MVAs are in the Latin American and Caribbean region, whereas India has the greatest rate of TBI-related injuries due to falls.[1] In the United States alone, more than 1.4 million people have a TBI every year, whereas annual estimates of sports-related concussions range from 1.6 to 3.8 million.[2] Concussion is defined as transient and immediate alteration in brain function, including alteration of mental status and level of consciousness, caused by a blow to the head.[3] In a broader sense, The American Academy of Neurology defines concussion as "a pathophysiologic disturbance in neurologic function characterized by clinical symptoms induced by biomechanical forces."[4] However, the definition of concussion still remains

Disclosures: The authors have nothing to disclose.
This work was supported by the DUNN Research Foundation.
[a] Department of Diagnostic and Interventional Imaging, The University of Texas Health Science Center, McGovern Medical School, 6431 Fannin Street, MSB 2.100, Houston, TX 77030, USA; [b] Department of Neurology, The University of Texas Health Science Center, McGovern Medical School, 6431 Fannin Street, Houston, TX 77030, USA; [c] Department of Physical Medicine and Rehabilitation, Baylor College of Medicine, Michael E. DeBakey VA Medical Center, 7200 Cambridge Street, Suite 9A, Houston, TX 77030, USA; [d] Department of Neurology, Baylor College of Medicine, Michael E. DeBakey VA Medical Center, 7200 Cambridge Street, Suite 9A, Houston, TX 77030, USA; [e] Department of Radiology, Baylor College of Medicine, Michael E. DeBakey VA Medical Center, 7200 Cambridge Street, Suite 9A, Houston, TX 77030, USA
* Corresponding author.
E-mail address: Khader.M.Hasan@uth.tmc.edu

controversial; it is sometimes applied differently in sports-related, emergency department, and military environments; and the terms *mild TBI* (mTBI) and *concussion* are often used interchangeably.[5]

The burden of mortality and morbidity associated with head trauma makes TBI a pressing public health and medical problem. Public health concerns about head trauma also relate to repeated impact to the head in recreational and professional sports, including ice hockey, soccer, football, martial arts, boxing, and other sports that may affect the normal development of the brain, especially in children, adolescents, and young adults. Repeated sports-related concussions (SRCs) at a young age may affect normal brain development and prevent recovery in some cases.[6] Although most patients who sustain SRCs recover quickly and are asymptomatic within a short amount of time, a notable minority of patients experience persistent symptoms after concussion, sometimes referred to as postconcussion syndrome.[7] SRCs have been associated with an increased risk for depression and memory problems,[8] chronic traumatic encephalopathy (CTE),[9] Alzheimer dementia,[10–12] Parkinson disease,[13] and cerebrovascular diseases, which may occur through decreases in cerebral blood flow and cerebral vascular reactivity[14] as well as other patho-mechanisms.

MECHANISMS OF INJURY

TBI-induced damage can be divided into injuries at macroscopic and microscopic levels (Fig. 1). Macroscopic injuries can be divided into primary

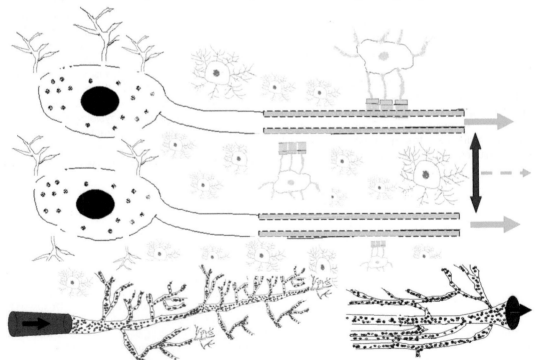

Axons/Myelin **(extra and** intra-axonal**)**

Blood Vessels "arterial/venous"

Neurons/Dendrites

Glia (Dendrocytes**/Astrocytes/Macrophages)**

Fig. 1. Common injury mechanisms in TBI. Secondary to injury, glial activation takes place to further exacerbate the axonal, neuronal, and myelin injury, including the arterial and venous system.

and secondary injuries. Primary injuries consist of diffuse axonal injury; cortical contusion; subcortical gray-matter injury; primary brainstem injuries; and epidural, subdural, subarachnoid, intraventricular, and intraparenchymal hemorrhages.[15–17] Secondary injuries consist of pressure necrosis secondary to brain displacement and herniation, territorial arterial infarction,[18] diffuse hypoxic injury, diffuse brain swelling, secondary hemorrhages, fatty embolism, or infection.[19,20] At the microscopic level, TBI may lead to hypoxia and oxidative stress,[21] excitotoxicity, inhibitory dysregulation, injury secondary to essential metabolites, altered ratios of n-acetylaspartate (NAA)/creatinine (Cr), NAA/choline and choline/Cr, inflammation and apoptosis.[22] It is still unclear whether and how much each of these injuries contribute to concussion or mTBI generally; the contribution of each of these mechanisms may vary with several factors, including the severity and circumstances of the injury as well as numerous host-related factors (eg, age, sex, and so forth).[23]

PROMISES OF MULTIMODAL NEUROIMAGING AND UTILITY IN CONCUSSION

In most cases of concussion, conventional computed tomography and MR imaging are normal and the diagnosis is made based on clinical assessment. Unavoidably, some cases remain undiagnosed, as their symptoms are subtle.[24] In addition, it remains difficult to predict outcomes based on initial clinical and imaging assessment. Advanced imaging technologies, using multimodal MR imaging, may be better at evaluating and predicting outcomes after concussion.[25] Multimodal imaging modality has the potential to go beyond diagnosis to include prognostication of the clinical course of concussion, establishing machine learning systems to discover noninvasive in vivo biomarkers, assessing the efficacy of existing pharmacologic and rehabilitative therapies, and guiding the development of new treatment modalities, such as noninvasive brain stimulations, robot-assisted rehabilitations, and brain-machine interfaces.[26]

Conventional MR imaging (cMR imaging) data typically use a single high spatial resolution volume (ie, isotropic 1 mm) for anatomic landmark identification, lesion localization (ie, T2-weighted [T2w]-fluid-attenuated inversion recovery [FLAIR]), and tissue segmentation (white matter, gray matter, and cerebrospinal fluid [CSF]) and parcellation (eg, entorhinal cortex, hippocampus) in order to derive measurement of the tissue volume, thickness, shape, and other morphometrics. Such measurements may be useful in determining regional patterns of relative vulnerability of brain tissue in both early and late phases after a TBI. Morphometrics have also been applied to examine how mild brain injury may disrupt typical development, interact with aging, or potentially accelerate change associated with neurodegeneration.[27,28] Multiple cMR imaging volumes may be coregistered and/or fused to improve the accuracy of abnormal tissue localization and normal-appearing tissue segmentation. Synthetic or derived composite volumes may also be obtained by simple algebraic operations to enhance tissue contrast, such as T1-weighted (T1w)/T2w ratio maps and T2w*FLAIR or other combination maps. Tissue attributes derived from these maps are generally referred to as macrostructural and include volume, surface area, gyrification, curvature, and cortical thickness. Free software tools used for tissue segmentation include FreeSurfer, Advanced Normalization Tools, and MRIcloud.[29]

Advanced MR imaging methods typically acquire multiple volumes (ie, multidimensional) by varying one or 2 image parameters (ie, repetition time [T_R], echo time [T_E], inversion time, diffusion gradient pulse weighting and orientation, velocity-encoding, magnetization transfer pulse frequency and strength, and so forth). These volumes are acquired with or without contrast while patients are at rest (eyes closed/open) or actively involved in a cognitive or sensory-motor task. In general, multidimensional MR imaging data are coregistered and modeled to provide regional quantitative maps or qMR imaging, which includes diffusion-based MR imaging (dMR imaging), perfusion-based MR imaging, functional MR imaging (fMR imaging), quantitative venography, susceptibility-weighted imaging/quantitative susceptibility mapping, magnetization transfer, and relaxometry. Relaxation-based methods have been used to infer water, myelin, and iron content. The measures derived from qMR imaging also include diffusivity, anisotropy, and relaxation rate. Blood or CSF-derived speed measures combined with area estimation provide volume or production rates and may also be related to intracranial pressure. Tissue attributes derived from these maps may be calibrated to provide core brain temperature, and white matter tissue orientation may be connected by fiber tracking methods.

Methods that use arterial spin labeling by continuous inversion of inflow blood may also be calibrated to infer regional cerebral blood flow. These methods may also be modeled using multi-compartments to estimate the regional cerebral blood volume. In the concussion literature, this method is shown to be possibly useful for explaining the neuroprotective regulation of cerebral blood flow in mTBI,[30] assessing functional abnormalities,[31] and detecting and tracking the longitudinal course of the underlying neurophysiologic recovery from concussions.[32]

Pathologic hallmarks of secondary injury, such as microedema, microbleeds, gliosis, demyelination, axonal loss, and perfusion penumbra, may not be directly measured; advanced models may be needed to address the shortcomings of the current clinical protocols. Previous pathologic studies have shown the accumulation of tau protein in concussions.[9] Some of the pathologic features of

CTE overlap with the accumulation of beta amyloid in Alzheimer's disease (AD). Advances in imaging methods, such as multiband, compressed sensing, and high field clinical scanners (ie, 7.0 T), promise to provide more pathology-specific models per unit scan time with improved spatial resolution. The 7.0-T MR imaging can accurately detect iron deposits within activated microglia, which may help shed light on the role of the immune system in AD pathogenesis.[33] Interestingly, T2 relaxation time at 7.0 T is associated with amyloid pathologic accumulation in animal models of AD.[34] It has been postulated that TBI may lead to plaque formation in the brain as suggested by nuclear medicine methods.[11] In the near future, advanced magnetic resonance methods may provide a noninvasive and more cost-effective alternative to PET imaging.

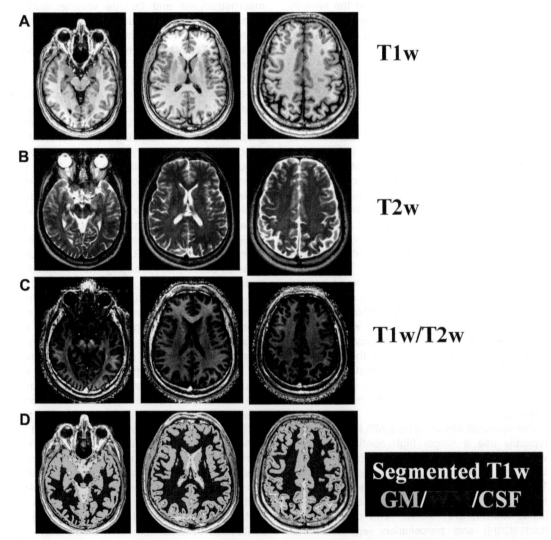

Fig. 2. T1w/T2w ratio and tissue segmentation maps derived from T1w. GM, gray matter; WM, white matter.

OVERVIEW OF MULTIMODAL ADVANCED IMAGING MODALITIES

In this section, the authors provide a short overview and pictorial display of basic contrast mechanisms that are used in MR imaging to localize and visualize injuries. The authors emphasize the value of using multimodal and multidimensional MR imaging methods to improve pathologic specificity. As an illustration of the use of multimodal MR imaging methods, the data were acquired from one healthy adult control. The data included high-resolution T1w, multi-echo T1w, T2w, and diffusion-weighted and perfusion-weighted maps via pulsed arterial spin labeling. Multimodal data were processed to obtain T1, T2, relaxation times, water content, and diffusion-derived maps as described elsewhere.[29] All maps were coregistered to the T1w data space. **Fig. 2** shows the T1w/T2w ratio and tissue segmentation maps derived from T1w. **Fig. 3** shows the T1, T2

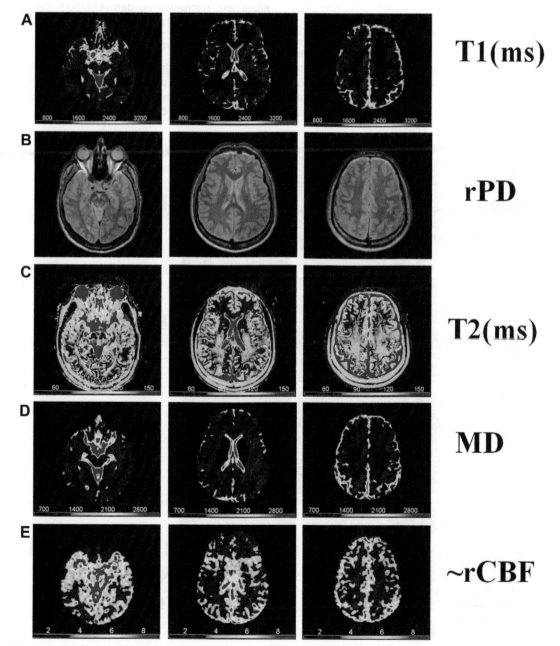

Fig. 3. T1, T2 relaxation time (in milliseconds) maps and relative water content proton density (rPD), mean diffusivity (MD) and regional cerebral blood flow (rCBF)/volume maps.

relaxation time maps and relative water content proton density (PD), mean diffusivity, and regional cerebral blood flow/volume maps. **Fig. 4** shows the utility of single tensor diffusion tensor imaging (DTI) to obtain fractional anisotropy, radial and axial diffusivity, in addition to tissue orientation. Note that iron-rich structures (ie, red nuclei) are not readily visible on T1w but are evident on taking the ratio map of T1w/T2w. The axial diffusivity is greater in compact white matter compared with gray matter.

T1-Weighted Contrast and T1 Relaxation Time

T_1 relaxation time is an intrinsic tissue parameter that may be a sensitive and early marker of pathology (ie, in trauma, multiple sclerosis, AD, and so forth). T_1 also depends on the temperature, regional blood flow, and extrinsic contrast agents (oxygen inhalation, iron oxide, gadolinium, and oxygen in CSF) that can alter its regional values. The values for blood, fat, muscle, and white and gray matter are different and depend on age and sex. The T_1 maps can also be helpful in tissue segmentation and partial volume modeling, as the parameter is independent from the tissue intensities. T1w maps are usually acquired with short T_E to minimize T2-relaxation effects. Hyperintensities on T1w images (ie, due to iron, oxygen, calcification, lipids) and hypointensities (eg, microedema, demyelination) can be interpreted using the optimized signal intensity:

$$S_{spoiled\_GE} \propto PD \times \exp\left(-\frac{T_E}{T_{2^*}}\right) \times \sqrt{\frac{T_R}{T_1}}$$

White matter has lower T1 values than gray matter because of the presence of greater myelin in white matter. However, it should be noted that in regions with reduced myelin, the iron content can

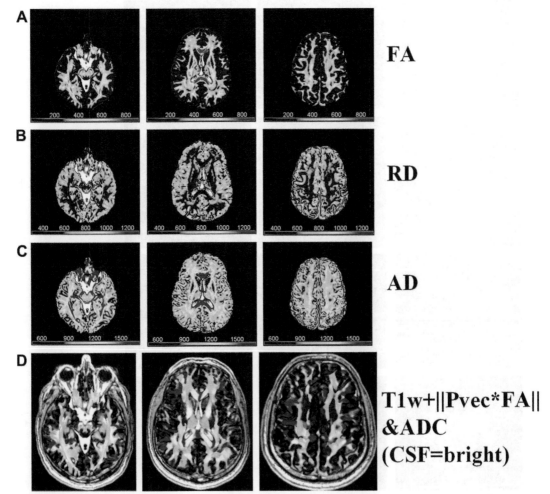

Fig. 4. The utility of single tensor DTI to obtain fractional anisotropy (FA), radial (RD) and axial diffusivity (AD) in addition to tissue orientation. ADC, apparent diffusion coefficient; Pvec, principal eigenvector modulated by FA.

be a confounder as it reduces T1. Mapping of the true T_1 and T_2 relaxation times and water content PD would provide more specific information compared with the signal intensity, which has PD and T_2 effects.

T2-Weighted Contrast and T2 Relaxation Time

The estimation of T_2 uses the spin-echo approach in which the signal at different T_ES are acquired and modeled using the nonexchanging multicompartment model:

$$S(T_E, T_R, T_1, T_2) = \sum_{i=1}^{Nc} PD_i * f(T_R, T_{1i}) \exp\left(-\frac{T_E}{T_{2i}}\right)$$

In general, the signal may originate from different compartments (ie, blood, myelin water, intracellular and extracellular water). Both relative water content and T_2 can be estimated for each compartment by changing T_E, keeping T_R, and all other temporal-spatial parameters fixed.

Diffusion-Weighted Contrast and Beyond

Diffusion-sensitized images are usually acquired with the spin echo approach using diffusion-gradient pulses with calibrated amplitude, duration, and separation to provide a controlled signal attenuation for a given diffusion pulse. The signal acquired may originate from random thermal diffusion, which can be free Gaussian, hindered or restricted non-Gaussian, and nonthermal diffusion originating from randomly distributes capillaries, or the so-called intravoxel incoherent motion (IVIM). The IVIM pseudodiffusion amounts to mapping the blood volume in the voxel and requires low b factors (ie, b <300 s/mm^{-2}). Gaussian diffusion modeling is usually adopted in single diffusion tensor imaging, which requires a minimum of 6 directions uniformly distributed over the unit hemisphere with the b factor approximately 1000 s/mm. The Gaussian model may also include free water (fw) in the extracellular space. Restricted diffusion has been shown to be best modeled with high b factors (ie, b >2000) using high order

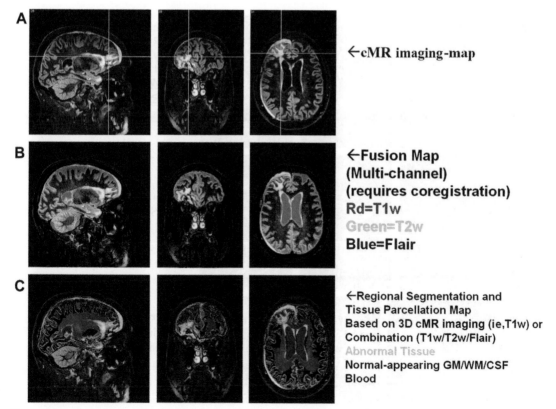

←cMR imaging-map

←Fusion Map
(Multi-channel)
(requires coregistration)
Rd=T1w
Green=T2w
Blue=Flair

←Regional Segmentation and
Tissue Parcellation Map
Based on 3D cMR imaging (ie,T1w) or
Combination (T1w/T2w/Flair)
Abnormal Tissue
Normal-appearing GM/WM/CSF
Blood

Fig. 5. The injury location along with subdural hematoma, diffuse axonal injury, and symmetric periventricular white matter hyperintensities that are age-related in this 74-year-old man with a history of sports-related repetitive head trauma as well as a fall. B, blue; G, green; GM, gray matter; R, red; WM, white matter.

tensors, diffusion kurtosis imaging (DKI), and neurite orientation dispersion and density imaging (NODDI). In general, a host of b factors and diffusion gradient pulses are acquired; the nonlinear model described later is used to fit the acquired data[35,36]:

Gradient Echo, Phase, and Susceptibility-Weighted Imaging

Signal-attenuation in gradient echo is influenced by dephasing and consequent signal losses due to field inhomogeneities that include external magnetic field B_0 and local magnetic susceptibility

$$S = S(0) * \left(f_{IVIM} * \exp(-bD_f) + fw * \exp(-ADC_{fw} * b) + (1 - f_{IVIM} - fw) * \exp\left(-b*ADC + (b*ADC)^2 * K/6 \right) \right)$$

where ADC is the apparent diffusion coefficient.

The recent application of multi-shell dMR imaging (ie, DKI, NODDI) to both animal and human mTBI show promising results to resolve astrogliosis[37,38] and mapping the fraction of water in the extra-axonal and intra-axonal compartments.[39–42]

effects. Conventional single compartment multi-gradient echo methods used magnitude data to map iron content via R2* = R2+R2' (R2: reversible, R2': irreversible) or magnetic field correlation.[43] The acquisition of both magnitude and phase using multi-gradient echoes in combination with local filter and dipole inversion methods has

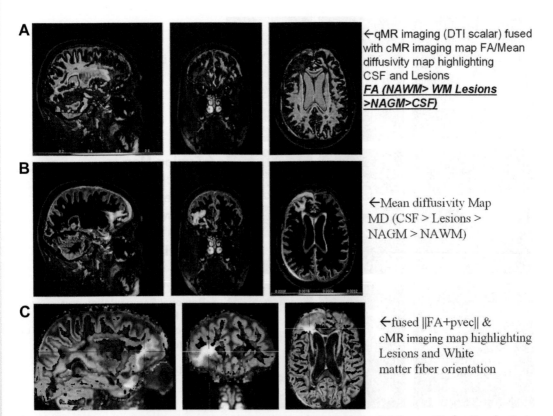

A ←qMR imaging (DTI scalar) fused with cMR imaging map FA/Mean diffusivity map highlighting CSF and Lesions **FA (NAWM> WM Lesions >NAGM>CSF)**

B ←Mean diffusivity Map MD (CSF > Lesions > NAGM > NAWM)

C ←fused ||FA+pvec|| & cMR imaging map highlighting Lesions and White matter fiber orientation

Fig. 6. The scalar and orientation maps derived from the DTI fused with the FLAIR map. FA, fractional anisotropy; MD, mean diffusivity; NAGM, normal-appearing gray matter; NAWM, normal-appearing white matter; pvec, principal eigenvector.

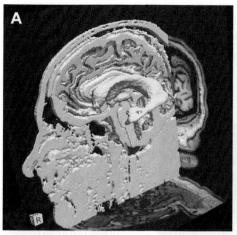
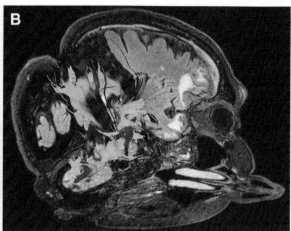

Fig. 7. A 3D illustration of sulcal and ventricular CSF *(yellow)* *(A)* and cerebello-cerebral pathways and motor-sensory pathways *(B)* in the authors' case.

enabled the mapping of veins, oxygenation state of blood, and the tissue diamagnetism and paramagnetism state that help in quantification of iron content, microbleeds, and hematomas.[44,45] Gradient echo methods are also routinely adopted in pulsed arterial spin labeling to estimate cerebral blood flow. The blood-oxygenation level dependent is used in the resting and active state fMR imaging and is shown to be useful in measuring the physiologic correlates of concussive symptoms.[46,47]

ILLUSTRATION OF THE APPLICATION OF QUANTITATIVE MR IMAGING TO TRAUMATIC BRAIN INJURY

To demonstrate the utility of multimodal MR imaging in TBI research, the authors describe a patient who sustained repeated sports-related brain injury and who also fell off a ladder, with impact to the right frontal lobe that caused a subdural hematoma (SDH). The data acquired included T1w, T2w, CSF fluid, and white matter–attenuated double inversion recovery, gradient echo, and DTI. Fig. 5 shows the injury location along with SDH, diffuse axonal injury (DAI), and symmetric periventricular white matter hyperintensities (WMH) that are age related (74 years old). The combination of multimodal images after registration provided clear tissue segmentation. Fig. 6 shows the scalar and orientation maps derived from the DTI fused with the FLAIR map. Note the extent of DAI that included right frontotemporal connections (ie, callosal forceps minor, uncinate fasciculus) that could explain his auditory-verbal memory issues as well as self-awareness of his deficits and limitations the authors have detected in their

clinical examination.[48] The data were processed further to show the 3-dimensional (3D) sulcal and ventricular CSF (Fig. 7A). The motor and sensory cortical and cerebellar pathways seem to be intact in this case (Fig. 7B). However, the cerebellum itself is interestingly affected in TBI as it sits in the posterior fossa, which is relatively smaller and has less CSF around it as a shock absorber.[11,49,50] Fig. 8 shows the WMH (red), DAI, and corpus callosum (white) with respect to the brainstem, hippocampus, and amygdala. The connections of these structures to the frontal cortex, shown in Fig. 9, will

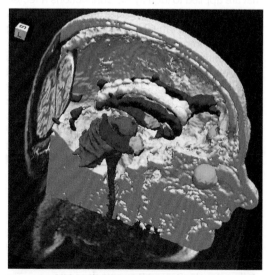

Fig. 8. White matter hyperintensities *(red)*, diffuse axonal injury *(bright red)*, corpus callosum *(white)* with respect to brainstem *(blue)*, hippocampus *(dark pink)* and amygdale *(light purple)*, and eyes *(green)*.

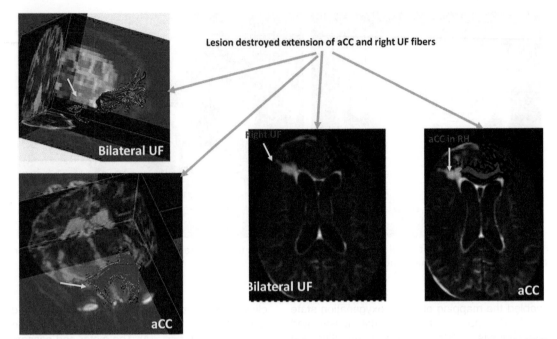

Fig. 9. Fiber tractography revealing affected right uncinate fasciculus (UF) and anterior corpus callosum (aCC) fibers in a 74-year-old subject. Extension of the tracts is damaged by the lesion in right anterior frontal regions. Both the right and left sides are illustrated for the comparison.

be monitored in a longitudinal follow-up of this patient.

SUMMARY

The authors present an overview of conventional and advanced multimodal MR imaging methods that are applied to identify the connections affected in TBI. The authors emphasize the value of using multimodal and multidimensional MR imaging methods to improve the pathologic specificity.[51–53] The potential utility of multimodal imaging provides improvements in diagnosis, predicting the clinical course of concussion and assessing the efficacy of existing and newly emerging pharmacologic and rehabilitative therapies.[54,55] Various pathologic hallmarks of primary and secondary injuries may not be directly measured, and advanced models may be needed to address the shortcomings of the current clinical protocols.

REFERENCES

1. Hyder AA, Wunderlich CA, Puvanachandra P, et al. The impact of traumatic brain injuries: a global perspective. NeuroRehabilitation 2007;22:341–53.
2. Langlois JA, Rutland-Brown W, Wald MM, et al. The epidemiology and impact of traumatic brain injury – a brief overview. J Head Trauma Rehabil 2006;21: 375–8.
3. Blyth BJ, Bazarian JJ. Traumatic alterations in consciousness: traumatic brain injury. Emerg Med Clin North Am 2010;28:571–94.
4. Giza CC, Kutcher JS, Ashwal S, et al. Summary of evidence-based guideline update: evaluation and management of concussion in sports: report of the Guideline Development Subcommittee of the American Academy of Neurology. Neurology 2013;80: 2250–7.
5. Harmon K, Drezner J, Gammons M, et al. American Medical Society for Sports Medicine position statement: concussion in sport. Br J Sports Med 2013; 47:15–26.
6. Terwilliger VK, Pratson L, Vaughan CG, et al. Additional post-concussion impact exposure may affect recovery in adolescent athletes. J Neurotrauma 2016;33(8):761–5.
7. Mannix R, Meehan WP III, Pascual-Leone A. Sports-related concussions — media, science and policy. Nat Rev Neurol 2016;12:486–90.
8. Guskiewicz KM, Marshall SW, Bailes J, et al. Recurrent concussion and risk of depression in retired professional football players. Med Sci Sports Exerc 2007;39:903–9.
9. McKee AC, Cantu RC, Nowinski CJ, et al. Chronic traumatic encephalopathy in athletes: progressive tauopathy after repetitive head injury. J Neuropathol Exp Neurol 2009;68(7):709–35.
10. Mielke MM, Savica R, Wiste HJ, et al. Head trauma and in vivo measures of amyloid and

neurodegeneration in a population-based study. Neurology 2014;82(1):70–6.

11. Scott G, Ramlackhansingh AF, Edison P, et al. Amyloid pathology and axonal injury after brain trauma. Neurology 2016;86(9):821–8.

12. Furst JA, Bigler ED. Amyloid plaques in TBI. Neurology 2016;86:798–9.

13. Harris MA, Shen H, Marion SA, et al. Head injuries and Parkinson's disease in a case-control study. Occup Environ Med 2013;70(12):839–44.

14. Ellis MJ, Ryner LN, Sobczyk O, et al. Neuroimaging assessment of cerebrovascular reactivity in concussion: current concepts, methodological considerations, and review of the literature. Front Neurol 2016;7:61.

15. Holbourn AHS. Mechanics of head injuries. Lancet 1943;2:438–41.

16. Holbourn AHS. The mechanics of brain injuries. Br Med Bull 1945;3:147–9.

17. Quillinan N, Herson PS, Traystman RJ. Neuropathophysiology of brain injury. Anesthesiol Clin 2016;34:453–64.

18. Siesjo BK. Basic mechanisms of traumatic brain damage. Ann Emerg Med 1993;22:959–69.

19. Gentry LR, Godersky JC, Thompson B. MR imaging of head trauma: review of the distribution and radiopathologic features of traumatic lesions. AJR Am J Roentgenol 1988;9:101–10.

20. Gentry LR, Thompson B, Godersky JC. Trauma to the corpus callosum: MR features. AJR Am J Roentgenol 1988;9:1129–38.

21. McIntosh TK, Smith DH, Meaney DF. Neuropathological sequelae of traumatic brain injury: relationship to neurochemical and biochemical mechanisms. Lab Invest 1996;74:315–42.

22. Van Horn JD, Bhattrai A, Irimia A. Multimodal imaging of neurometabolic pathology due to traumatic brain injury. Trends Neurosci 2017;40(1):39–59 [pii: S0166-2236(16)30144-8].

23. Clark MD, Asken BM, Marshall SW, et al. Descriptive characteristics of concussions in National Football League games, 2010-2011 to 2013-2014. Am J Sports Med 2017. https://doi.org/10.1177/0363546516677793.

24. Narayana PA, Yu X, Hasan KM, et al. Multi-modal MRI of mild traumatic brain injury. Neuroimage Clin 2014;7:87–97.

25. Wilde EA, Bouix S, Tate DF, et al. Advanced neuroimaging applied to veterans and service personnel with traumatic brain injury: state of the art and potential benefits. Brain Imaging Behav 2015;9:367–402.

26. Bigler ED. Systems biology, neuroimaging, neuropsychology, neuroconnectivity and traumatic brain injury. Front Syst Neurosci 2016;10:55.

27. Mayer AR, Ling JM, Dodd AB, et al. A longitudinal assessment of structural and chemical alterations in mixed martial arts fighters. J Neurotrauma 2015; 32(22):1759–67.

28. Meier TB, Bellgowan PS, Bergamino M, et al. Thinner cortex in collegiate football players with, but not without, a self-reported history of concussion. J Neurotrauma 2016;33(4):330–8.

29. Hasan KM, Walimuni IS, Abid H, et al. Multimodal quantitative magnetic resonance imaging of thalamic development and aging across the human lifespan: implications to neurodegeneration in multiple sclerosis. J Neurosci 2011;31(46):16826–32.

30. Doshi H, Wiseman N, Liu J, et al. Cerebral hemodynamic changes of mild traumatic brain injury at the acute stage. PLoS One 2015;10(2):e0118061.

31. Wang Y, West JD, Bailey JN, et al. Decreased cerebral blood flow in chronic pediatric mild TBI: an MRI perfusion study. Dev Neuropsychol 2015;40(1):40–4.

32. Wang Y, Nelson LD, LaRoche AA, et al. Cerebral blood flow alterations in acute sport-related concussion. J Neurotrauma 2016;33:1227–36.

33. Ali R, Goubran M, Choudhri O, et al. Seven-tesla MRI and neuroimaging biomarkers for Alzheimer's disease. Neurosurg Focus 2015;39(5):E4.

34. Li L, Wang XY, Gao FB, et al. Magnetic resonance T2 relaxation time at 7 tesla associated with amyloid B pathology and age in a double-transgenic mouse model of Alzheimer's disease. Neurosci Lett 2016; 610:92–7.

35. Assaf Y, Holokovsky A, Berman E, et al. Diffusion and perfusion magnetic resonance imaging following closed head injury in rats. J Neurotrauma 1999;16(12):1165–76.

36. Iima M, Le Bihan D. Clinical intravoxel incoherent motion and diffusion MR imaging: past, present, and future. Radiology 2016;278:13–32.

37. Budde MD, Janes L, Gold E, et al. The contribution of gliosis to diffusion tensor anisotropy and tractography following traumatic brain injury: validation in the rat using Fourier analysis of stained tissue sections. Brain 2011;134(Pt 8):2248–60.

38. Zhuo J, Xu S, Proctor JL, et al. Diffusion kurtosis as an in vivo imaging marker for reactive astrogliosis in traumatic brain injury. Neuroimage 2012;59:467–77.

39. Stokum JA, Sours C, Zhuo J, et al. A longitudinal evaluation of diffusion kurtosis imaging in patients with mild traumatic brain injury. Brain Inj 2015; 29(1):47–57.

40. Davenport EM, Apkarian K, Whitlow CT, et al. Abnormalities in diffusional kurtosis metrics related to head impact exposure in a season of high school varsity football. J Neurotrauma 2016;33(23):2133–46.

41. Grossman EJ, Kirov II, Gonen O, et al. N-acetyl-aspartate levels correlate with intra-axonal compartment parameters from diffusion MRI. Neuroimage 2015;118:334–43.

42. Mayer AR, Ling JM, Dodd AB, et al. A prospective microstructure imaging study in mixed-martial artists using geometric measures and diffusion tensor imaging: methods and findings. Brain Imaging Behav 2016. https://doi.org/10.1007/s11682-016-9546-1.

43. Raz E, Jensen JH, Ge Y, et al. Brain iron quantification in mild traumatic brain injury: a magnetic field correlation study. AJNR Am J Neuroradiol 2011;32: 1851–6.

44. Liu J, Xia S, Hanks R, et al. Susceptibility weighted imaging and mapping of micro-hemorrhages and major deep veins after traumatic brain injury. J Neurotrauma 2016;33:10–21.

45. Trifan G, Gattu R, Haacke EM, et al. MR imaging findings in mild traumatic brain injury with persistent neurological impairment. Magn Reson Imaging 2016;37:243–51.

46. Mayer AR, Bellgowan PS, Hanlon FM. Functional magnetic resonance imaging of mild traumatic brain injury. Neurosci Biobehav Rev 2015;49:8–18.

47. Wu X, Kirov II, Gonen O, et al. MR imaging applications in mild traumatic brain injury: an imaging update. Radiology 2016;279:693–707.

48. Levine B, Black SE, Cabeza R, et al. Episodic memory and the self in a case of isolated retrograde amnesia. Brain 1998;121(Pt 10):1951–73.

49. Spanos GK, Wilde EA, Bigler ED, et al. Cerebellar atrophy after moderate to severe traumatic brain injury. AJNR Am J Neuroradiol 2007;28:537–42.

50. Magnoni S, Mac Donald CL, Esparza TJ, et al. Quantitative assessments of traumatic axonal injury in human brain: concordance of microdialysis and advanced MRI. Brain 2015;138(Pt 8): 2263–77.

51. Wright AD, Jarrett M, Vavasour I, et al. Myelin water fraction is transiently reduced after a single mild traumatic brain injury–A prospective cohort study in collegiate hockey players. PLoS One 2016;11(2): e0150215.

52. Holleran L, Kim JH, Gangolli M, et al. Axonal disruption in white matter underlying cortical sulcus tau pathology in chronic traumatic encephalopathy. Acta Neuropathol 2017;133(3):367–80.

53. Ghajari M, Hellyer PJ, Sharp DJ. Computational modelling of traumatic brain injury predicts the location of chronic traumatic encephalopathy pathology. Brain 2017;140(Pt 2):333–43.

54. Wintermark M, Sanelli PC, Anzai Y, et al. Imaging evidence and recommendations for traumatic brain injury: advanced neuro- and neurovascular imaging techniques. AJNR Am J Neuroradiol 2015;36:E1–11.

55. McCrory P, Meeuwisse WH, Aubry M, et al. Consensus statement on concussion in sport: the 4th International Conference on Concussion in Sport, Zurich, November 2012. J Athl Train 2013; 48:554–75.

Imaging of Concussion in Young Athletes

Jeffrey P. Guenette, MD[a,b], Martha E. Shenton, PhD[a,b,c,d], Inga K. Koerte, MD[b,d,e],*

KEYWORDS

- Concussion • Mild traumatic brain injury • Head trauma • Sports • Pediatrics • MR imaging
- Diffusion tensor imaging • Susceptibility-weighted imaging

KEY POINTS

- Routine clinical imaging is typically not indicated in sports-related concussion.
- Per the American Association of Neurology and the American Medical Society of Sports Medicine guidelines, in concussion, imaging should only be performed if there are concerns regarding skull fracture, intracranial hemorrhage, or other intracranial disorders based on clinical examination.
- There are many studies that may lead to important diagnostic and prognostic neuroimaging biomarkers that will assist in the diagnosis of brain alterations associated with concussion and that indicate those who are most at risk for adverse outcomes. This information will become available clinically over the next decade.
- Screening for clinical neuroimaging biomarkers will likely become important in ensuring adequate positive and negative predictive values and to maintain cost-effectiveness.
- Although some neuroimaging examinations may be appropriate in the acute phase of injury, many are likely to be more appropriate in the subacute or chronic phases, and the timing of examinations depends on clinical presentation.

INTRODUCTION

Concussion, also known as mild traumatic brain injury (mTBI), is a clinical syndrome characterized by an immediate but transient alteration in brain function, generally caused by a blunt force. In young athletes, the cause is typically a direct blow to the head. The American Academy of Neurology and the American Medical Society for Sports Medicine guidelines currently indicate that there is no role for routine clinical imaging in sports-related concussion given that the findings are typically negative.[1,2] However, many new and emerging imaging techniques show potential diagnostic and prognostic value.

EPIDEMIOLOGY

Half of pediatric emergency department visits for concussion are sports related.[3] Specifically, more than 170,000 children aged 19 years or younger are seen annually for sports and recreation–related traumatic brain injury in the United States.[4] Further, more than 62,000 cases of concussion occur annually in high school varsity athletes, 60% of which occur in football players.[5]

Disclosures: J.P. Guenette has nothing to disclose. M.E. Shenton is supported by NIH 1U01NS093334-01 and VA Merit Award I01 RX00928. I.K. Koerte is supported by NIH R01NS100952.
a Department of Radiology, Brigham and Women's Hospital, Harvard Medical School, 75 Francis Street, Boston, MA 02115, USA; b Psychiatry Neuroimaging Laboratory, Department of Psychiatry, Brigham and Women's Hospital, Harvard Medical School, 1249 Boylston Street, Boston, MA 02215, USA; c VA Boston Healthcare System, Brockton Division, 940 Belmont Street, Brockton, MA 02301, USA; d Department of Psychiatry, Massachusetts General Hospital, Harvard Medical School, 55 Fruit Street, Boston, MA 02114, USA; e Department of Child and Adolescent Psychiatry, Psychosomatic, and Psychotherapy, Ludwig-Maximilian-Universität, Nußbaumstr 5a, Munich 80336, Germany
* Corresponding author. Psychiatry Neuroimaging Laboratory, 1249 Boylston Street, Boston, MA 02215.
E-mail address: ikoerte@bwh.harvard.edu

Moreover, concussion comprises nearly 9% of reported high school athletic injuries and 6% of collegiate athletic injuries,[6] and there is evidence that sports-related concussion is substantially underreported. For example, amateur male hockey players report approximately 14 times more concussions than official reports of such injury suggest.[7] The most common symptom of concussion is headache, which occurs in 93.4% of concussed high school athletes, whereas loss of consciousness occurs 4.6% of the time.[8]

Reported rates of concussion in high school sports increased 4.2-fold between 1997 to 1998 and 2007 to 2008,[9] and this increase corresponds with a similar increased rate of concussion-related emergency department visits, which has doubled in children 8 to 13 years old and tripled in children 14 to 19 years old in the United States over this same time period. Of note, this increase is despite an overall decline in participation in organized team sports.[3] A similar rate of increase in emergency department visits for concussion has also been reported by the US Centers for Disease Control and Prevention for the years 2001 to 2009.[4] The activities most associated with youth emergency department visits for concussion are bicycling, football, playground activities, basketball, and soccer.[4] In addition, more than 10% of youth emergency department visits for concussion are related to horseback riding, ice skating, golfing, all-terrain vehicle riding, and tobogganing/sledding.[4]

SEX DIFFERENCES IN CONCUSSION

Although more than 70% of emergency department patients with sports and recreation–related concussion visits are male,[4] high school girls experience twice the rate of concussion as boys participating in similar sports.[9] Even more concerning is that female high school and collegiate athletes who sustain a concussion experience more frequent cognitive impairment, greater declines in simple and complex reaction times relative to preseason baseline levels, and also more postconcussion symptoms compared with male athletes.[10] A study of children hospitalized after concussion also reports more severe symptoms in girls than in boys at presentation.[11] Similar findings have been identified in a study of female soccer players who performed worse on computer-based neuropsychiatric testing after concussion than did male players,[12] and in a neuroimaging study of female athletes who had more severe white matter abnormalities at 6 months postconcussion than did male athletes.[13]

CONSIDERATIONS REGARDING TIMING OF IMAGING

Based on physical examination, clinical anatomic imaging is performed in the acute setting if skull fracture or hemorrhage is suspected. Although cognitive function typically returns to baseline in 5 to 7 days,[14] in one study of 416 children and adolescents with concussion, 29.3% had postconcussion symptoms at 3 months, and missed more than 1 week of school on average.[15] Similarly, in another study of 190 children, almost 25% experienced headache, 20% fatigue, and 20% longer thinking times at 1 month, with average sleep disturbances lasting 16 days.[16] Given that these symptoms are measured on a timeline of weeks to months, it is important to develop imaging biomarkers to identify the acute or subacute phase to determine whether or not this information will have value in predicting outcome (prognosis). Thus imaging examinations performed in the chronic phase at 1 month to 3 months are more likely to reveal alterations in the brain that may be useful in predicting which patients are most likely to have prolonged postconcussive symptoms or even permanent cognitive deficits.

OBJECTIVE OF THIS ARTICLE

Research on neuroimaging of concussion in young athletes is currently focused on identifying highly sensitive and quantitative measures of early concussion diagnosis and on accurate prognosis. The goal of these efforts is to identify imaging markers that can be used as biomarkers that provide important clinical information, including an individual's risk for prolonged postconcussive symptoms, risk for long-term cognitive deficits, and an appropriate time interval before return to play. This article discusses the results of advanced imaging techniques that are currently being used in neuroimaging research in youth concussion, with an emphasis on those techniques that may soon be incorporated into the clinical evaluation of concussed young athletes.

Normal Anatomy and Imaging Technique

Traditional clinical anatomic imaging
The American Academy of Neurology guidelines recommend conventional clinical neuroimaging in the setting of suspected concussion in those patients who have loss of consciousness, posttraumatic amnesia, persistent Glasgow Coma Scale score less than 15, focal neurologic deficit, evidence of skull fracture on examination, or signs of clinical deterioration.[1] Neuroimaging in this

context is to rule out more severe traumatic brain injury. Similarly, the American Medical Society of Sports medicine guidelines recommend traditional clinical neuroimaging only when there is concern for intracranial hemorrhage.[2]

Computed tomography (CT) imaging is the first-line imaging in head injury:

- CT generally has higher spatial resolution than magnetic resonance (MR) imaging
- CT is more sensitive than MR imaging for the evaluation of the osseous calvarium, provides exceptional sensitivity for hemorrhage, and makes possible the detection of foreign objects inside the calvarium that would preclude MR imaging
- CT is generally cheaper, more readily available, and much faster than MR imaging

CT findings in moderate to severe brain trauma include skull base fracture, epidural hemorrhage related to laceration of the middle meningeal artery from an adjacent fracture (**Fig. 1**), and subarachnoid hemorrhage or cerebral contusion related to brain compression and friction along the rough inner calvarial surface (**Fig. 2**). However, the use of CT includes the risk of exposure to ionizing radiation and it lacks sensitivity for detecting diffuse white matter injury and subtle structural brain alterations. MR imaging is far more sensitive for detecting diffuse axonal injury, which is the most common injury observed in concussion (**Fig. 3**).

Considerations regarding patient selection for imaging

Advanced imaging techniques are nonetheless time consuming and expensive. Screening is thus important in considering its use in the evaluation of concussion. For example, screening based on a history of prior concussion may be appropriate given that high school football players with prior concussion have a greater risk of future concussion.[17] High school athletes with a history of prior concussion are also more likely to experience on-field loss of consciousness, anterograde amnesia, and confusion,[18] and they perform more poorly on memory testing, attention, and concentration following a new concussion than do athletes experiencing their first concussion.[12,19] Similarly, screening of athletes with academic problems may be appropriate to evaluate for prior concussion particularly given that high school athletes with a history of 2 or more concussions often perform similarly on baseline measures of concentration and attention to those recently concussed.[20] Screening based on duration of on-field symptoms may also be appropriate given that high school athletes with on-field mental status changes for more than 5 minutes have

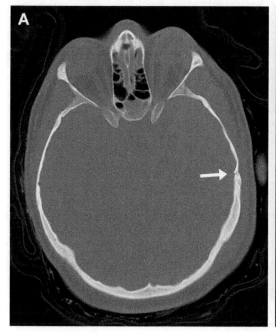
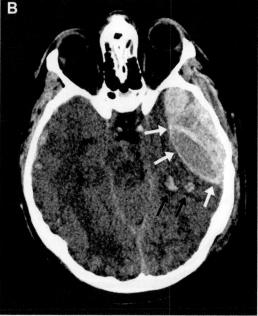

Fig. 1. A 23-year-old man ejected from motor vehicle. (*A*) Axial CT image bone windows shows a temporal bone fracture (*arrow*) in the region of the middle meningeal artery. (*B*) Axial CT image in soft tissue windows at the same level as *A* shows an associated large epidural hemorrhage (*white arrows*). Small foci of intraparenchymal hemorrhage are also visible (*black arrows*). (*Courtesy of* Liangge Hsu, MD, Brigham and Women's Hospital.)

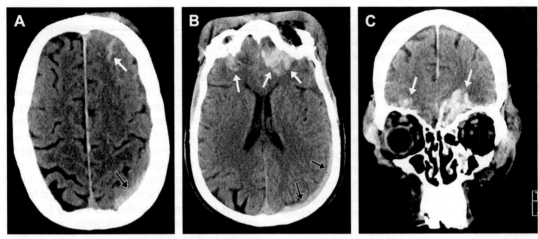

Fig. 2. A 46-year-old man after a 4.5-m (15 feet) fall from a roof. (*A*) Axial CT image in soft tissue windows shows a left frontal subarachnoid hemorrhage (*white arrow*) and left parietal subdural hemorrhage (*black arrow*). A left frontal subgaleal hematoma is also present. (*B*) Axial CT image in soft tissue windows, more inferior than that in *A*, shows bifrontal brain contusions (*white arrows*) and left parietal subdural hemorrhage (*black arrows*). (*C*) Coronal CT image in soft tissue windows shows the same bifrontal contusions (*white arrows*) clearly located along the floor of the anterior cranial fossa, which is a common location because of sudden traumatic compression of the brain in this region.

longer-lasting postconcussion symptoms and memory decline than those with a shorter durations of symptoms.[21] In addition, screening based on age may be appropriate given that high school athletes show prolonged memory dysfunction following concussion compared with college athletes.[22] At present, known clinical markers associated with longer time to recovery, such as

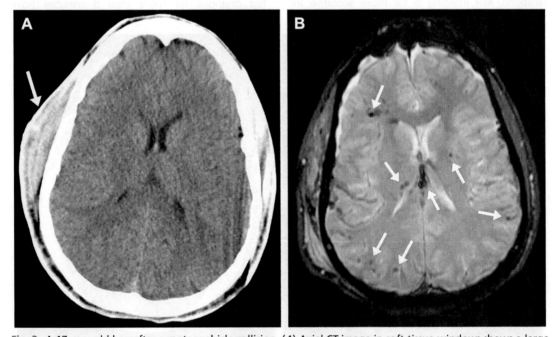

Fig. 3. A 17-year-old boy after a motor vehicle collision. (*A*) Axial CT image in soft tissue windows shows a large right subgaleal hematoma (*arrow*) without any evident intracranial abnormality. (*B*) Axial gradient-recall echo (GRE) MR image in a similar plane shows foci of susceptibility artifact (*arrows*), presumed to represent microhemorrhage, scattered along the gray-white junction, in the right thalamus, in the left putamen, and in the fornix body. Susceptibility-weighted imaging has replaced GRE at our institution in most routine imaging protocols. (*Courtesy of* Liangge Hsu, MD, Brigham and Women's Hospital.)

self-reported cognitive decline, reaction time, and migraine symptoms,[23] may also play a role in patient selection for screening using imaging.

Two imaging protocols are discussed here: the first is used in the clinical setting at Boston Children's Hospital; the second is an example of a protocol used in research studies to evaluate for subtle alterations following concussion in young athletes (Box 1).

Imaging Findings/Pathology

Clinical anatomic imaging

As noted previously, routine clinical imaging in concussion is discouraged by both the American Academy of Neurology and the American Medical Society for Sports Medicine because of low diagnostic yield.[1,2] For example, in a study of 151 youth patients with sports-related concussion, 8 patients had abnormal neuroimaging findings.[24] Of note, this subset of patients was likely self-selected for greater-than-average symptoms given that many individuals with concussion never seek medical care.

Structural quantitative high-resolution magnetic resonance imaging

High-resolution, three-dimensional (3D), T1-weighted MR imaging sequences provide very good anatomic detail of the brain. Using a tool such as 3D Slicer (Surgical Planning Laboratory, Brigham and Women's Hospital, Boston, MA), regions of interest within the brain can be manually segmented or parcellated. Further, tools such as FreeSurfer (Athinoula A. Martinos Center for Biomedical Imaging, Charlestown, MA) and FMRIB Software Library (Analysis Group, Oxford Centre for Functional MR imaging of the Brain, Oxford, United Kingdom) also allow automated brain segmentation and parcellation (Fig. 4).

Cortical atrophy has been observed in pediatric patients with concussion 4 months postinjury.[25] Similarly, children with moderate/severe traumatic brain injury may evince widespread cortical thinning 3 years postinjury.[26] Cortical thickness is also associated with memory performance.[26] Also of note, there seems to be an association between accelerated decline in cortical thickness with age and a history of repetitive concussive and subconcussive mTBI.[27,28] As for deep gray matter volumes, a study of college football players with a history of prior clinician-diagnosed concussion showed smaller hippocampal volumes in players with a history of concussion compared with those without a history of concussion.[29] There is also an apparent association between repeated head trauma and smaller thalamus size.[30]

Box 1
Imaging protocols

Noncontrast clinical MR imaging protocol for concussion in young athletes

- Three-dimensional (3D) T1-weighted magnetization prepared rapid gradient echo (recovery time [TR] = 1520 milliseconds, echo time [TE] = 2.27 milliseconds, voxel size = 0.86 mm sagittal × 1 mm axial × 1 mm coronal, acquisition matrix = 256 × 256)

- Axial T2 spin echo (TR = 4300 milliseconds, TE = 89 milliseconds, slice thickness = 2.5 mm, acquisition matrix = 325 × 512)

- Axial T2 fluid-attenuated inversion recovery (FLAIR; TR = 8000 milliseconds, TE = 137 milliseconds, slice thickness = 4 mm, acquisition matrix = 288 × 320)

- Axial susceptibility-weighted imaging (SWI; TR = 27 milliseconds, TE = 20 milliseconds, slice thickness = 1.25 mm, acquisition matrix = 232 × 256)

- Diffusion tensor imaging (DTI) with tractography and trace diffusion-weighted imaging (directions = 35, b = 1000, TR = 9500 milliseconds, TE = 88 milliseconds, slice thickness = 2 mm, acquisition matrix = 128 × 128)

Research protocol in our laboratory for mTBI

- 3D T1-weighted magnetization prepared rapid gradient echo (TR = 1800 milliseconds, TE = 3.36 milliseconds, voxel size = 1 × 1 × 1 mm, acquisition matrix = 256 × 256, flip angle = 7°)

- 3D T2-weighted FLAIR (TR = 3200 milliseconds, TE = 456 milliseconds, voxel size = 1 × 1 × 1 mm, acquisition matrix = 256 × 256)

- DTI (directions = 64, b = 3000, TR = 13,600 milliseconds, TE = 111 milliseconds, slice thickness = 2 mm, acquisition matrix = 256 × 256)

- SWI (TR = 30 milliseconds, TE = 23 milliseconds, voxel size = 1 × 1 × 1 mm, acquisition matrix = 256 × 256)

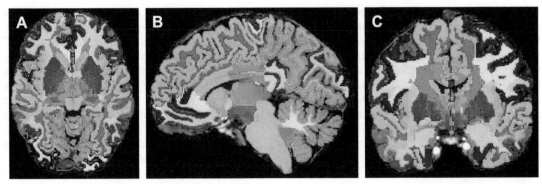

Fig. 4. (*A*) Axial, (*B*) sagittal, and (*C*) coronal images of the brain with automatic segmentation label maps generated by FreeSurfer superimposed on T1-weighted high-resolution MR images.

Tissue architecture diffusion tensor imaging

Diffusion tensor imaging (DTI) is an MR method that measures diffusion of water molecules (see review by Basser and Jones[31]). Diffusion measures can be calculated based on brain regions of interest and they can be used to analyze white matter fiber tracts (**Fig. 5**). The physiologic interpretation of DTI measures is well described.[32,33] The most commonly reported diffusion measure is fractional anisotropy (FA). FA describes the likelihood of directionality of the diffusion of water. Diffusion MR imaging is a particularly promising technique for evaluating the subtle structural brain alterations following concussion, such as diffuse axonal injury, noted previously as the most common injury after concussion. Diffuse axonal injury can be identified and quantified using diffusion MR imaging. In the last few years, many studies have been published using diffusion MR imaging in mTBI (see Shenton and colleagues[34] for a comprehensive review).

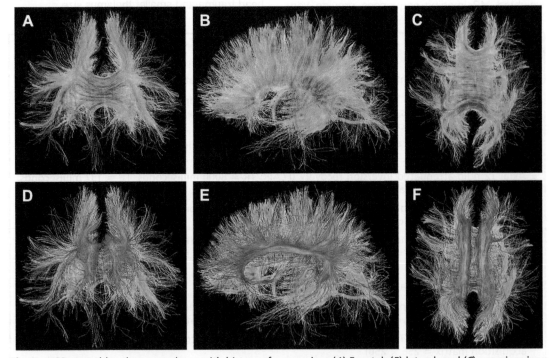

Fig. 5. A 22-year-old male soccer player with history of concussion. (*A*) Frontal, (*B*) lateral, and (*C*) superior views of corpus callosum white matter fiber tracts generated with 2-tensor tractography from diffusion-weighted images. The interhemispheric traversing fibers are particularly well shown on the frontal and superior views. (*D*) Frontal, (*E*) lateral, and (*F*) superior views of corpus callosum (warm colors) and cingulate gyri (cyan spectrum) white matter fiber tracts generated with 2-tensor tractography from diffusion-weighted images. Quantitative measures of the tracts are used to identify subtle white matter abnormalities not visible on conventional imaging.

In adolescents, DTI abnormalities have been identified in the first week postconcussion.[35] Moreover, white matter DTI abnormalities that are present in the first week postconcussion have been shown to persist at 6 months postconcussion in adult athletes.[36] In young adult hockey players with a history of concussion, increased FA levels in the left genu and in the anterior corona radiata are observed compared with teammates with no history of concussion, suggesting regional white matter microstructural injury following concussion.[37] Similarly, regional diffusion abnormalities are observed in female athletes in the corpus callosum at 6 months postconcussion,[13] and also in other white matter regions in pediatric patients 4 months postconcussion, despite partial normalization in cognitive tests.[25] Taken together, these findings suggest that concussion-related white matter injuries may still be evident as clinical symptoms begin to resolve, or they may continue with persistent postconcussive symptoms.

Susceptibility-weighted imaging of microhemorrhage

Susceptibility-weighted imaging (SWI) is MR imaging designed to enhance the contrast between tissues with different magnetic susceptibilities.[38] SWI is particularly useful in evaluating paramagnetic properties that are present in deoxyhemoglobin and hemosiderin, which are the blood products of hemorrhage. SWI is sensitive for detecting brain lesions at all TBI severity levels in children[39] and is more sensitive than CT and traditional clinical MR imaging for the detection of traumatic lesions in children following TBI.[40] Moreover, SWI is also useful in predicting cognitive outcomes in the initial stages postinjury, when the number and volume of microhemorrhages in children with mTBI, and with more severe TBI, have been shown to correlate with neurologic outcome.[39] A proposed new quantitative technique has shown possible detection of microhemorrhage in collegiate hockey players over a single season.[41] SWI measures are thus likely to be most useful for acute injury to detect microbleeds, which often resolve over time.

Regional blood flow imaging

Dynamic susceptibility contrast (DSC) MR imaging, also known as dynamic contrast-enhanced (DCE) MR imaging, makes it possible to measure regional cerebral blood flow.[42] DSC/DCE imaging is not frequently used in studies of concussion because of the need for administration of intravenous contrast material. However, noninvasive alternatives, such as arterial spin labeling (ASL) and phase contrast imaging, are being investigated in concussion.[43–45]

A phase contrast imaging study of pediatric sports-related concussion showed cerebral blood flow alterations immediately following concussive trauma, with a trend for blood flow patterns to return toward baseline values at 14 days (27%) and 30 days (64%).[46] Similar findings have been described in the acute phase with regional blood flow reductions correlating with postconcussive symptoms in studies with ASL MR imaging.[47,48] Abnormal regional cerebral blood flow has also been shown in chronic pediatric mTBI[49] and in adults 2 years following concussion.[50] However, further studies are needed to determine whether noncontrast enhanced regional blood flow imaging may inform prognosis following concussion in youth athletes.

Functional magnetic resonance imaging

Blood oxygenation level–dependent (BOLD) MR imaging can be used as a proxy to evaluate cerebral blood flow changes in active brain regions.[51] Accordingly, functional MR (fMR) imaging can evaluate brain region activation during the performance of specific tasks. It can also be used to evaluate regions of brain activation in the state of relaxed consciousness (also known as resting state) in order to evaluate regions associated with cognitive abilities and attention.[52,53]

Abnormalities in the default mode network, which is assumed to be a network of interacting brain regions with highly correlated activity, can be seen acutely in college varsity athletes in the first week following concussion.[54] Focal abnormalities in the prefrontal cortex can be seen in male athletes with postconcussive symptoms.[55] Moreover, there is evidence that fMR imaging may be predictive of recovery in concussed high school athletes.[56] Long-term abnormalities in fMR imaging studies have also been identified in the chronic stages following concussion.[57,58] Taken together, fMR imaging may be sensitive in assessing alterations in brain function and connectivity following concussion. However, to be useful in the clinical setting, analysis techniques would need to reveal patient-specific alterations in addition to comparisons on a group level.

Metabolic imaging

MR spectroscopy (MRS) imaging quantifies human tissue metabolites in vivo. A recent comprehensive review of MRS in brain imaging describes the clinical utility of MRS.[59] Although MRS studies of adults with mTBI have suggested decreased regional axonal viability,[60] the only study on sports-related concussion in youth did not observe any N-acetylaspartate (neuron marker) or choline (cell membrane marker) abnormalities.[46] Further studies are needed to determine the efficacy of these measures in concussion.

PET and single-photon emission CT (SPECT) are performed by injecting a radioactive isotope bound to a metabolic tracer agent. The resolution of PET and SPECT is inferior to that of CT and MR imaging, which is problematic when trying to identify subtle changes as are expected in concussion. Moreover, radiotracer production and handling are expensive and involve intravenous injection of ionizing radiation, making PET and SPECT studies in young athletes generally not feasible at this time.

Current concerns regarding imaging of sports-related concussion

In addition to avoiding unnecessary radiation from CT,[1,2] cost also needs to be considered. The high costs per identified imaging abnormality when using conventional neuroimaging to evaluate concussion[61] reflect the lack of sensitivity of conventional imaging techniques for the detection of subtle brain alterations (mentioned earlier). Until advanced imaging techniques become available that show efficacy in evaluating concussion and the trajectory of recovery from concussion, the American Association of Neurology and American Medical Society for Sports Medicine guidelines should be followed. In addition, screening tools to identify those patients at risk for prolonged postconcussive symptoms should be developed.

Further, postconcussive syndrome is a heterogeneous disorder and is therefore difficult to study scientifically and also difficult to assess clinically because many symptoms overlap with other disorders such as depression and posttraumatic stress disorder.[62]

In addition, research studies often rely on group statistics, but mean and median group values in imaging studies may not capture pathologic processes that may occur in different locations. More objective radiological evidence is needed, which may have prognostic value in determining who is at risk for developing prolonged postconcussive symptoms. A method comparing concussed patients with a normative atlas has been proposed,[63] as has a statistical method called wild bootstrapping,[64] both of which attempt to identify patient-specific abnormalities. However, much more research is needed in this area to develop these methods for use in the clinic.

Diagnostic Criteria (List)

The diagnosis of concussion remains clinical at this time. Nonetheless, advanced imaging features offer radiological evidence that may soon support early diagnosis and provide prognostic information as well as monitor the efficacy of future treatments.

Differential Diagnosis (List/Callout Box)

There is no current radiological evidence that provides a differential diagnosis of concussion, because concussion is a clinical diagnosis based on an associated head trauma. In most cases, routine clinical CT or MR imaging do not reveal any abnormalities. However, future studies are needed to identify concussion-specific imaging markers so as to provide radiological and not just clinical evidence of concussion. Advanced MR techniques are likely to become available in the clinic in the near future, which will be useful for concussion diagnosis prognosis, and likely also for the monitoring of treatment efficacy as treatments become available for those patients who are most likely to experience persistent postconcussive symptoms.

What Referring Physicians Need to Know (List)

- Routine clinical imaging is typically not indicated in sports-related concussion.
- Per American Association of Neurology and American Medical Society of Sports Medicine guidelines, imaging should only be performed in concussion when there are concerns for skull fracture, intracranial hemorrhage, or other intracranial disorders based on physical examination.
- Potential diagnostic and prognostic neuroimaging biomarkers of concussion and adverse outcomes are being studied and may become clinically available over the next decade.
- Screening for clinical neuroimaging biomarkers are likely to be essential to ensure adequate positive and negative predictive values and to maintain cost-effectiveness.
- Although some neuroimaging biomarkers may be appropriate in the acute phase of injury, many are likely to be more appropriate in the subacute or chronic phases and timing will depend on the clinical concern.

SUMMARY

Potential diagnostic and prognostic neuroimaging biomarkers of concussion in young athletes are currently being investigated and may become available in the near future for integration into routine clinical imaging. Replication of preliminary results and the development of techniques to quantify imaging abnormalities on an individual basis, as opposed to group comparisons, are the next steps toward clinical implementation. The authors believe that the most promising approaches include a personalized, patient-specific profile of injuries that can be derived from multimodal neuroimaging. Accordingly, given the increasing number of reported sports-related concussions annually, neuroimaging biomarkers that provide critical information at an appropriate time interval before return to school and return to play, and based on the individual's risk for prolonged postconcussive symptoms as well as on long-term cognitive deficits, would have a substantial impact on the routine clinical management of sports-related concussion.

REFERENCES

1. Giza CC, Kutcher JS, Ashwal S, et al. Summary of evidence-based guideline update: evaluation and management of concussion in sports: report of the Guideline Development Subcommittee of the American Academy of Neurology. Neurology 2013; 80(24):2250–7.
2. Harmon KG, Drezner J, Gammons M, et al. American Medical Society for Sports Medicine position statement: concussion in sport. Clin J Sport Med 2013;23(1):1–18.
3. Bakhos LL, Lockhart GR, Myers R, et al. Emergency department visits for concussion in young child athletes. Pediatrics 2010;126(3):E550–6.
4. Centers for Disease Control and Prevention. Nonfatal traumatic brain injuries related to sports and recreation activities among persons aged ≤19 years — United States, 2001–2009. MMWR Morb Mortal Wkly Rep 2011;60(39):1337–42.
5. Powell JW, Barber-Foss KD. Traumatic brain injury in high school athletes. JAMA 1999;282(10):958–63.
6. Gessel LM, Fields SK, Collins CL, et al. Concussions among united states high school and collegiate athletes. J Athl Train 2007;42(4):495–503.
7. Williamson IJS, Goodman D. Converging evidence for the under-reporting of concussions in youth ice hockey. Br J Sports Med 2006;40(2):128–32.
8. Meehan WP, d'Hemecourt P, Comstock RD. High school concussions in the 2008-2009 academic year mechanism, symptoms, and management. Am J Sports Med 2010;38(12):2405–9.
9. Lincoln AE, Caswell SV, Almquist JL, et al. Trends in concussion incidence in high school sports a prospective 11-year study. Am J Sports Med 2011; 39(5):958–63.
10. Broshek DK, Kaushik T, Freeman JR, et al. Sex differences in outcome following sports-related concussion. J Neurosurg 2005;102(5):856–63.
11. Blinman TA, Houseknecht E, Snyder C, et al. Post-concussive symptoms in hospitalized pediatric patients after mild traumatic brain injury. J Pediatr Surg 2009;44(6):1223–8.
12. Colvin AC, Mullen J, Lovell MR, et al. The role of concussion history and gender in recovery from soccer-related concussion. Am J Sports Med 2009; 37(9):1699–704.
13. Chamard E, Lefebvre G, Lassonde M, et al. Long-term abnormalities in the corpus callosum of female concussed athletes. J Neurotrauma 2016;33(13): 1220–6.
14. McCrea M, Guskiewicz KM, Marshall SW, et al. Acute effects and recovery time following concussion in collegiate football players - The NCAA Concussion Study. JAMA 2003;290(19):2556–63.
15. Babcock L, Byczkowski T, Wade SL, et al. Predicting postconcussion syndrome after mild traumatic brain injury in children and adolescents who present to the emergency department. JAMA Pediatr 2013;167(2): 156–61.
16. Eisenberg MA, Meehan WP, Mannix R. Duration and course of post-concussive symptoms. Pediatrics 2014;133(6):999–1006.
17. Schulz MR, Marshall SW, Mueller FO, et al. Incidence and risk factors for concussion in high school athletes, North Carolina, 1996-1999. Am J Epidemiol 2004;160(10):937–44.
18. Collins MW, Lovell MR, Iverson GL, et al. Cumulative effects of concussion in high school athletes. Neurosurgery 2002;51(5):1175–9.
19. Iverson GL, Gaetz M, Lovell MR, et al. Cumulative effects of concussion in amateur athletes. Brain Inj 2004;18(5):433–43.
20. Moser RS, Schatz P, Jordan BD. Prolonged effects of concussion in high school athletes. Neurosurgery 2005;57(2):300–6.
21. Lovell MR, Collins MW, Iverson GL, et al. Recovery from mild concussion in high school athletes. J Neurosurg 2003;98(2):296–301.
22. Field M, Collins MW, Lovell MR, et al. Does age play a role in recovery from sports-related concussion? A comparison of high school and collegiate athletes. J Pediatr 2003;142(5):546–53.
23. Lau B, Lovell MR, Collins MW, et al. Neurocognitive and symptom predictors of recovery in high school athletes. Clin J Sport Med 2009;19(3):216–21.
24. Ellis MJ, Leiter J, Hall T, et al. Neuroimaging findings in pediatric sports-related concussion. J Neurosurg Pediatr 2015;16(3):241–7.
25. Mayer AR, Hanlon FM, Ling JM. Gray matter abnormalities in pediatric mild traumatic brain injury. J Neurotrauma 2015;32(10):723–30.
26. Merkley TL, Bigler ED, Wilde EA, et al. Diffuse changes in cortical thickness in pediatric moderate-to-severe traumatic brain injury. J Neurotrauma 2008;25(11):1343–5.

27. Tremblay S, De Beaumont L, Henry LC, et al. Sports concussions and aging: a neuroimaging investigation. Cereb Cortex 2013;23(5):1159–66.

28. Koerte IK, Mayinger M, Muehlmann M, et al. Cortical thinning in former professional soccer players. Brain Imaging Behav 2016;10(3):792–8.

29. Singh R, Meier TB, Kuplicki R, et al. Relationship of collegiate football experience and concussion with hippocampal volume and cognitive outcomes. JAMA 2014;311(18):1883–8.

30. Bernick C, Banks SJ, Shin W, et al. Repeated head trauma is associated with smaller thalamic volumes and slower processing speed: the Professional Fighters' Brain Health Study. Br J Sports Med 2015;49(15):1007–11.

31. Basser PJ, Jones DK. Diffusion-tensor MRI: theory, experimental design and data analysis - a technical review. NMR Biomed 2002;15(7–8):456–67.

32. Basser PJ, Pierpaoli C. Microstructural and physiological features of tissues elucidated by quantitative-diffusion-tensor MRI. J Magn Reson B 1996;111(3):209–19.

33. Wheeler-Kingshott CAM, Cercignani M. About "axial" and "radial" diffusivities. Magn Reson Med 2009;61(5):1255–60.

34. Shenton ME, Hamoda HM, Schneiderman JS, et al. A review of magnetic resonance imaging and diffusion tensor imaging findings in mild traumatic brain injury. Brain Imaging Behav 2012;6(2):137–92.

35. Chu Z, Wilde EA, Hunter JV, et al. Voxel-based analysis of diffusion tensor imaging in mild traumatic brain injury in adolescents. AJNR Am J Neuroradiol 2010;31(2):340–6.

36. Henry LC, Tremblay J, Tremblay S, et al. Acute and chronic changes in diffusivity measures after sports concussion. J Neurotrauma 2011;28(10):2049–59.

37. Orr CA, Albaugh MD, Watts R, et al. Neuroimaging biomarkers of a history of concussion observed in asymptomatic young athletes. J Neurotrauma 2016;33(9):803–10.

38. Haacke EM, Xu Y, Cheng YCN, et al. Susceptibility weighted imaging (SWI). Magn Reson Med 2004;52(3):612–8.

39. Beauchamp MH, Beare R, Ditchfield M, et al. Susceptibility weighted imaging and its relationship to outcome after pediatric traumatic brain injury. Cortex 2013;49(2):591–8.

40. Beauchamp MH, Ditchfield M, Babl FE, et al. Detecting traumatic brain lesions in children: CT versus MRI versus susceptibility weighted imaging (SWI). J Neurotrauma 2011;28(6):915–27.

41. Helmer KG, Pasternak O, Fredman E, et al. Hockey concussion education project, part 1. Susceptibility-weighted imaging study in male and female ice hockey players over a single season. J Neurosurg 2014;120(4):864–72.

42. Conturo TE, Akbudak E, Kotys MS, et al. Arterial input functions for dynamic susceptibility contrast MRI: requirements and signal options. J Magn Reson Imaging 2005;22(6):697–703.

43. Williams DS, Detre JA, Leigh JS, et al. Magnetic resonance imaging of perfusion using spin inversion of arterial water. Proc Natl Acad Sci U S A 1992;89(1):212–6.

44. Spilt A, Box FMA, van der Geest RJ, et al. Reproducibility of total cerebral blood flow measurements using phase contrast magnetic resonance imaging. J Magn Reson Imaging 2002;16(1):1–5.

45. Haller S, Zaharchuk G, Thomas DL, et al. Arterial spin labeling perfusion of the brain: emerging clinical applications. Radiology 2016;281(2):337–56.

46. Maugans TA, Farley C, Altaye M, et al. Pediatric sports-related concussion produces cerebral blood flow alterations. Pediatrics 2012;129(1):28–37.

47. Peng SP, Li YN, Liu J, et al. Pulsed arterial spin labeling effectively and dynamically observes changes in cerebral blood flow after mild traumatic brain injury. Neural Regen Res 2016;11(2):257–61.

48. Lin CM, Tseng YC, Hsu HL, et al. Arterial spin labeling perfusion study in the patients with subacute mild traumatic brain injury. PLoS One 2016;11(2): e0149109.

49. Wang Y, West JD, Bailey JN, et al. Decreased cerebral blood flow in chronic pediatric mild TBI: an MRI perfusion study. Dev Neuropsychol 2015;40(1):40–4.

50. Ge Y, Patel MB, Chen Q, et al. Assessment of thalamic perfusion in patients with mild traumatic brain injury by true FISP arterial spin labelling MR imaging at 3T. Brain Inj 2009;23(7):666–74.

51. Vitte E, Derosier C, Caritu Y, et al. Activation of the hippocampal formation by vestibular stimulation: a functional magnetic resonance imaging study. Exp Brain Res 1996;112(3):523–6.

52. Hampson M, Driesen NR, Skudlarski P, et al. Brain connectivity related to working memory performance. J Neurosci 2006;26(51):13338–43.

53. Kelly AM, Uddin LQ, Biswal BB, et al. Competition between functional brain networks mediates behavioral variability. NeuroImage 2008;39(1):527–37.

54. Militana AR, Donahue MJ, Sills AK, et al. Alterations in default-mode network connectivity may be influenced by cerebrovascular changes within 1 week of sports related concussion in college varsity athletes: a pilot study. Brain Imaging Behav 2016;10(2):559–68.

55. Chen JK, Johnston KM, Collie A, et al. A validation of the post concussion symptom scale in the assessment of complex concussion using cognitive testing and functional MRI. J Neurol Neurosurg Psychiatry 2007;78(11):1231–8.

56. Lovell MR, Pardini JE, Welling J, et al. Functional brain abnormalities are related to clinical recovery

and time to return-to-play in athletes. Neurosurgery 2007;61(2):352–9.

57. Sinopoli KJ, Chen JK, Wells G, et al. Imaging "Brain Strain" in youth athletes with mild traumatic brain injury during dual-task performance. J Neurotrauma 2014;31(22):1843–59.

58. Dettwiler A, Murugavel M, Putukian M, et al. Persistent differences in patterns of brain activation after sports-related concussion: a longitudinal functional magnetic resonance imaging study. J Neurotrauma 2014;31(2):180–8.

59. Oz G, Alger JR, Barker PB, et al. Clinical proton MR spectroscopy in central nervous system disorders. Radiology 2014;270(3):658–79.

60. Lin AP, Liao HJ, Merugumala SK, et al. Metabolic imaging of mild traumatic brain injury. Brain Imaging Behav 2012;6(2):208–23.

61. Morgan CD, Zuckerman SL, King LE, et al. Post-concussion syndrome (PCS) in a youth population: defining the diagnostic value and cost-utility of brain imaging. Childs Nerv Syst 2015;31(12): 2305–9.

62. Parker RS. Recommendations for the revision of DSM-IV diagnostic categories for co-morbid post-traumatic stress disorder and traumatic brain injury. NeuroRehabilitation 2002;17(2):131–43.

63. Bouix S, Pasternak O, Rathi Y, et al. Increased gray matter diffusion anisotropy in patients with persistent post-concussive symptoms following mild traumatic brain injury. PLoS One 2013;8(6):e66205.

64. Bazarian JJ, Zhu T, Blyth B, et al. Subject-specific changes in brain white matter on diffusion tensor imaging after sports-related concussion. Magn Reson Imaging 2012;30(2):171–80.

Perfusion Imaging in Acute Traumatic Brain Injury

David B. Douglas, MD[a,b], Ruchir Chaudhari, MD[a],
Jason M. Zhao, MD, PhD[b], James Gullo, MD[b],
Jared Kirkland, MD[b], Pamela K. Douglas, PhD[c],
Ely Wolin, MD[b], James Walroth, MD[b],
Max Wintermark, MD, MBA[a,*]

KEYWORDS

- Concussion • Traumatic brain injury • TBI • Perfusion

KEY POINTS

- Noncontrast computed tomography (CT) scan is the most appropriate initial neuroimaging study for a moderate to severe closed head injury.
- Perfusion CT has a higher sensitivity for detecting cerebral contusions than noncontrast CT examinations.
- Future research in perfusion imaging may improve the diagnosis, prognosis, and management of acute traumatic brain injury.

INTRODUCTION

Traumatic brain injury (TBI) is a major health care issue affecting 1.7 million people, hospitalizing 275,000 people and resulting in 52,000 deaths annually in the United States, and the incidence of emergency room visits related to TBI is increasing.[1–3] It is estimated that 3.2 million people are living with long-term disability from TBI.[4] The most common causes of TBI include motor vehicle accidents, falls, sports-related injury, and assault in the civilian population,[1–3] and explosion-related injury in the military.[5] Neuroimaging plays a key role in the diagnosis, treatment, and prognosis of TBI.

The American College of Radiology has provided appropriateness criteria to help referring physicians make the most appropriate decisions on imaging examinations. As an example, for a moderate or severe acute closed head injury (Glasgow Coma Scale <13), the most appropriate initial neuroimaging study is a noncontrast computed tomography (CT) scan.[6] A noncontrast CT scan can diagnose injuries, such as an epidural hematoma, that

Disclosures: The views expressed in this article are those of the authors and do not reflect the official policy or position of the US Government, the Department of Defense, or the Department of the Air Force. The animals involved in this study were procured, maintained, and used in accordance with the Laboratory Animal Welfare Act of 1966, as amended, and the Guide for the Care and Use of Laboratory Animals, National Research Council. The work reported herein was performed under United States Air Force Surgeon General approved Clinical Investigation Number FDG20160006A.
[a] Department of Neuroradiology, Stanford University Medical Center, 300 Pasteur Drive, Room S047, Stanford, CA 94305-5105, USA; [b] Department of Radiology, David Grant Medical Center, 101 Bodin Circle, Travis Air Force Base, CA 94535, USA; [c] Institute for Simulation and Training, University of Central Florida, 3100 Technology Parkway, Orlando, FL 32826, USA
* Corresponding author. Department of Neuroradiology, Stanford University Medical Center, 300 Pasteur Drive, Room S047, Stanford, CA 94305-5105.
E-mail address: mwinterm@stanford.edu

require emergent neurosurgical intervention. However, there are limitations associated with noncontrast CT scans. For example, early CT scans have been found to underestimate the size of parenchymal contusions.[7] For this reason, short-interval follow-up CT scans may be beneficial. In addition, early conventional noncontrast CT imaging does not show secondary ischemic changes related to cerebral edema and intracranial hypertension, which are responsible for nearly half of TBI-related deaths after admission.[8]

In recent years, neuroimaging has advanced beyond structural imaging to functional tissue characterization including cerebral perfusion. Perfusion is physiologically defined as the flow of blood per unit volume of tissue. The term tissue emphasizes that this specifically means capillary blood flow. Perfusion imaging is commonly used in clinical practice in the setting of stroke because it has the ability to distinguish normally perfused cerebral parenchyma from ischemic penumbra from infarcted tissue.[9–12] Recently, perfusion neuroimaging techniques have been explored in TBI to determine and characterize potential perfusion neuroimaging biomarkers to aid in diagnosis, treatment, and prognosis. Following TBI, it is thought that alterations in the cerebrovascular parameters may lead to secondary injuries.[13] The ability to improve clinical outcomes following TBI may rely on the ability to detect potentially salvageable tissue known as traumatic penumbra and secondary ischemic events.[14–16] This article reviews perfusion imaging techniques in TBI, including bolus perfusion CT (PCT), bolus perfusion MR imaging, arterial spin labeling (ASL) perfusion MR imaging, and stable xenon PCT. This article concludes with a discussion of future research techniques.

PERFUSION IMAGING IN COMPUTED TOMOGRAPHY
Introduction

The underlying basis for PCT is conservation of flow. In order to measure flow, a nondiffusible tracer (ie, an agent that remains in the vasculature) is administered intravenously. Bolus perfusion imaging is performed on a multidetector CT scanner in the axial plane typically with a 4 mL/s contrast injection rate.

With regard to image processing, the PCT images are used to create time-enhancement curves registered to each pixel in the data set. From the time-enhancement curves, processing software can generate key parameters, including regional cerebral blood volume (rCBV), mean transit time (MTT), and regional cerebral blood flow (rCBF),

which have been validated to stable xenon CT (Xe-CT).[17]

The cerebral blood volume (CBV) map is calculated from the area under the time-enhancement curves and represents the blood volume within the arterioles and venules of a given parenchymal tissue volume with units of milliliters of blood per 100 g of brain tissue. The MTT represents the average time that it takes for blood to flow from the arterial input through the brain tissue and to the venous drainage, and has units of seconds. MTT is calculated by a mathematical process called deconvolution.[18–20] The MTT requires a reference arterial input function (AIF), which commonly uses a region of interest drawn around the anterior cerebral artery. Time to peak is the time from the arrival of contrast into the AIF to the peak of the time-enhancement curve for each voxel. The time of maximum concentration (T_{max}) is calculated from the time to peak, with $T_{max} = 0$ for normal perfused tissue without delay.[21] In addition, cerebral blood flow (CBF) is the volume of blood flowing through a given volume of brain tissue over a certain time period and has units of milliliters of blood per 100 g of brain tissue per minute (**Fig. 1**).

The central volume principle describes the relationship between a compartment volume, blood flow through the compartment, and the mean transit time through the compartment.[12] According to the central volume principle, the MTT is equal to the rCBV divided by the rCBF.[22] The cerebral parenchyma viability is completely dependent on CBF. Alterations in CBF can influence electrical and metabolic neuronal activity. Cerebral autoregulation plays a role in ensuring that there is adequate CBF despite alterations in systemic pressure.

Bolus Computed Tomography Perfusion Imaging Applied to Acute Traumatic Brain Injury

Wintermark and colleagues[23] explored PCT on admission CT scans and found perfusion abnormalities associated with juxtadural collections, cerebral edema, and intracranial hypertension. In the Wintermark and colleagues[23] study, which included 48 patients who had cerebral contusions diagnosed on delayed follow-up imaging, 19 of the 48 contusions were seen on the initial noncontrast CT images (sensitivity of 39.6%) and 42 of the 48 were seen on the PCT images (sensitivity of 87.5%). The 42 perfusion abnormalities were noted to occur in the same location as the contusion on delayed CT. The difference in the sensitivity of noncontrast CT and PCT was statistically significant ($P<.001$). The specificity of

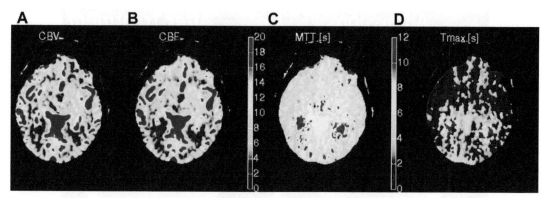

Fig. 1. Normal CT perfusion images showing (*A*) rCBV, (*B*) rCBF, (*C*) MTT, and (*D*) T$_{max}$.

perfusion defects for cerebral contusion in the setting of severe trauma was 93.9%.[23] In the setting of cerebral contusions, focal cortical-subcortical perfusion abnormalities of increased MTT, decreased rCBF, and decreased rCBV were noted (**Fig. 2**).[23] Areas of vasogenic edema could either show increased perfusion or decreased perfusion and areas of cytotoxic edema showed decreased perfusion.[23] In the setting of juxtadural collections, decreased rCBF was found to be decreased in the immediate vicinity of epidural hematomas (**Fig. 3**).[23,24] In Wintermark and colleagues'[23] study, increased MTT, decreased rCBF, and decreased rCBV were observed in the setting of intracranial hypertension (**Fig. 4**).[23]

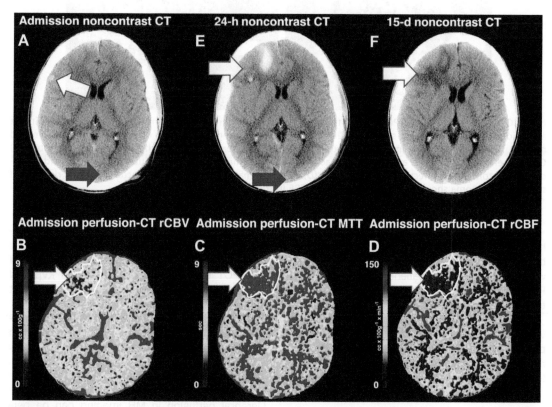

Fig. 2. Contrast-enhanced and PCT images from a patient with severe TBI. (*A*) Noncontrast CT at admission shows a small hemorrhagic contusion in the right frontal lobe (*arrow*). Admission PCT images show a large territory of decreased rCBV (*B*), increased MTT (*C*), and decreased rCBF (*D*). Follow-up noncontrast CT at 24 hours (*E*) shows increased areas of hemorrhagic contusion in the right frontal lobe where the perfusion abnormality was seen. Follow-up noncontrast CT at 15 days (*F*) shows evolving hemorrhagic contusion and encephalomalacia in the right frontal lobe, which corresponds with the same distribution that is seen on the PCT.

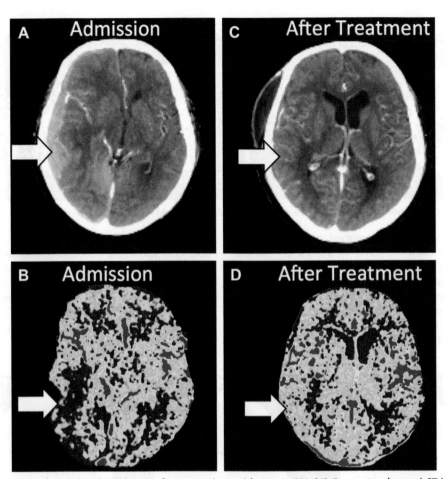

Fig. 3. Contrast-enhanced and PCT images from a patient with severe TBI. (*A*) Contrast-enhanced CT imaging at admission shows a right-sided subdural hematoma (*arrow*) causing mass effect on the underlying brain and midline shift. (*B*) rCBF PCT imaging at admission shows decreased rCBF in the right temporal lobe. (*C*) Contrast-enhanced CT image after surgical evacuation of the hematoma shows resolution of the right-sided subdural hematoma, mass effect, and midline shift. (*D*) rCBF PCT imaging after surgical evacuation of the right-sided subdural hematoma shows normalization of the rCBF in the right temporal lobe.

Even with no visible intracranial injury on admission head CT, perfusion imaging with acute reductions in blood flow and blood volume are associated with worse outcomes.[24] In patients with severe TBI, PCT showed additional information in 60% of patients and altered management in 10% of patients.[25]

Areas of hypodensity on CT may be necrotic or viable and PCT may help distinguish between these possibilities.[26] PCT also provides insight into the cerebral vascular autoregulation, which may be used to guide therapy and monitor treatment efficiency.[26]

Challenges of Computed Tomography Perfusion Imaging in Acute Traumatic Brain Injury

One of the key challenges is the radiation dose that accompanies PCT. Radiation safety is of paramount importance and the aim of every institution should be to keep radiation dose as low as reasonably achievable. It has been suggested that PCT should be performed at 80 kVp and 100 mAs, to maximize the contrast enhancement and decrease the radiation dose.[27]

Another risk of PCT is the intravenous administration of contrast material, which can result in renal impairment or allergic reaction.

PERFUSION IMAGING IN MR IMAGING

Cerebral perfusion in MR imaging can be performed via 2 main approaches. The first method is through the exogenous intravenous administration of a nondiffusible contrast agent, such as gadolinium-based contrast agents.[28] The second method is through endogenous magnetic labeling

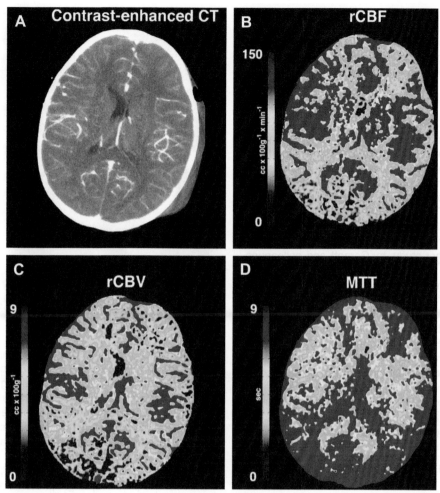

Fig. 4. Contrast-enhanced and PCT images of a case of TBI with intracranial hypertension. The contrast enhanced CT (*A*) showed left-sided scalp hematoma. The rCBF (*B*) and rCBV (*C*) trended toward lower values, especially in the occipital lobes. The MTT (*D*) showed significantly higher values, reflecting altered cerebral autoregulation after TBI.

of arterial blood water as a diffusible flow tracer in ASL MR perfusion.[28]

BOLUS PERFUSION MR IMAGING
Introduction

In bolus perfusion MR imaging, also known as bolus tracking, an exogenous, nondiffusible contrast agent, such as a gadolinium-based contrast agent, is administered intravenously.[28] Within nondiffusible brain perfusion imaging there are 2 main categories: dynamic susceptibility weighted contrast (DSC) and dynamic contrast enhancement (DCE) imaging.[28]

In DSC, the gadolinium-chelate bolus causes transient decrease in signal intensity by the T2* effect of the contrast bolus during the initial pass through the vasculature.[28] This effect results in

decreased signal with increased contrast. A typical DSC bolus MR imaging sequence requires an intravenous injection rate of a gadolinium-based contrast agent of approximately 4 mL/s. A gradient-echo echo-planar sequence is performed with a total scan time of approximately 1 to 2 minutes during the injection of the contrast bolus.

In DCE, the gadolinium-chelated bolus causes T1 shortening within the blood pool and within any area that accumulates because of leakage outside of vessels. This T1 shortening results in increased signal with increased contrast.[28]

As previously discussed in DSC imaging, as the contrast bolus arrives, a transient signal decrease in T2* occurs. A plot of the contrast concentration curve over time, C(t), is called the time-concentration curve. A plot of the signal intensity over time is called the time-intensity curve. Note that the time-intensity curves in bolus perfusion MR imaging are logarithmically related to the time-concentration curves.[11] The rest of the calculations in bolus perfusion MR imaging are similar to those described earlier for PCT.

Bolus MR Perfusion Imaging Applied to Traumatic Brain Injury

In one study of TBI in a military population by Liu and colleagues,[29] voxelwise analysis of rCBF maps showed scattered perfusion defects in the cerebellum, cingulate gyrus, cuneus, and temporal gyrus in patients with TBI compared with normal controls. This study also showed correlations of the perfusion defects with verbal memory, reaction time, and self-reported stress.[29]

In another study, by Garnett and colleagues,[13] DSC was performed in 18 patients with subacute TBI (mean of 10 days following TBI). Six of the 18 patients had visible contusions on conventional MR imaging and each of these 6 patients had significantly reduced rCBV in the contused regions.[13] Five of the 18 patients had reduced rCBV in areas where a contusion was not identified on conventional imaging. These 5 patients were not more significantly injured than the remaining patients but had worse clinical outcomes.[13]

Challenges of Bolus MR Perfusion Imaging in Acute Traumatic Brain Injury

In general, performing an MR imaging scan in the setting of trauma can be difficult. Patients may be hemodynamically unstable. Because MR imaging scans are inherently long, patients may not be able to be cleared for MR imaging. Furthermore, patients with trauma may be unable to complete the MR imaging safety questionnaire because of unconscious state or may have known contraindications to MR imaging. For this reason, MR imaging in the setting of trauma is inherently challenging.

ARTERIAL SPIN LABELING MR IMAGING
Introduction

ASL is a noninvasive MR imaging technique that offers quantitative information on the CBF and perfusion (Fig. 5). The technique was successfully implemented for the first time in a rat CBF model by Williams and colleagues.[30] ASL uses radiofrequency (RF) pulses to invert water proton spins by 180° in the regions inferior to the brain slice of interest. A labeling image is acquired as these tagged protons flow along the cerebral vasculature and enter the slice; another control image is sequentially obtained in the same slice but without the RF inversion; the difference between the labeling and

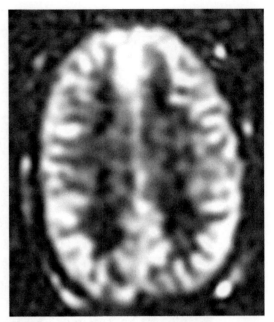

Fig. 5. Normal noncontrast ASL sequence.

control images is used to create a map of CBF and perfusion as highlighted by endogenous proton spins. ASL signal is affected by physiologic parameters, including labeling efficiency, arterial blood T1 and T2, blood transport time through vessels and tissue, and magnetization transfer effects.[30–33]

ASL-based CBF measurements have been validated against traditional radiotracer perfusion techniques, including hexamethylpropylene amine oxime (HMPAO) single-photon emission CT (SPECT),[34] PET,[35] and Xe-CT.[36] This versatile technique also generates reproducible results that have been confirmed by multicenter clinical trials.[37] ASL has multiple attractive features compared with other perfusion imaging techniques. ASL uses endogenous water protons as opposed to contrast agents and avoids radiation exposure, making it ideal for imaging in pediatric and pregnant patients.[38] In addition, ASL modeling allows quantification of absolute CBF, which can be used to perform longitudinal studies, as well as comparison studies between different MR imaging scanners.

Arterial Spin Labeling MR Imaging Applied to Traumatic Brain Injury

Since its inception, ASL has been widely used in various clinical applications, including stroke, arteriovenous malformations, dementia, epilepsy, central nervous system tumors, and infections.[39] ASL has also been used in several TBI perfusion studies in animals and human subjects.

In 2002, Kochanek and colleagues[40] performed one of the pioneer animal experiments using ASL to investigate the effect of TBI on CBF in rats after controlled cortical impact (CCI). They measured T1 relaxation times in a slice through the plane of injury using continuous ASL imaging at 1 year after injury and found an 80% reduction in CBF in the regions of interest immediately next to the lesion when comparing CCI subjects with sham-surgery subjects.[40] Despite significant tissue loss in both ipsilateral and contralateral hemispheres, they did not find widespread reduction in CBF, which they attributed to remodeling of the brain to maintain constant CBF outside the primary lesion.[40]

The chronic effects of mild TBI (mTBI) on regional CBF and neuropsychological function were studied by Ge and colleagues[41] using a True FISP ASL labeling sequence on a 3-T scanner. Comparing 21 patients with clinical diagnosis of mTBI with healthy controls, the investigators found a statistically significant decrease in CBF in patients with mTBI in bilateral thalami and caudate nuclei but not in putamen or frontal white matter. Moreover, the CBF changes were positively correlated with the changes in processing, response speed, memory, verbal fluency, and executive function of the subjects with mTBI. This remarkable study correlated quantitative CBF measurements with neuropsychological impairment, making an important connection between brain physiology and the common clinical symptoms of patients.

Kim and colleagues[42] studied the resting CBF in 27 patients with chronic moderate to severe TBI and compared them with matched controls. They discovered a global, nonuniform hypoperfusion with prominent regional decreases in the thalami and posterior cingulate gyri, where the greatest volume losses also occurred. They suggested that structural lesions contribute to chronic CBF changes; in particular, signal loss in posterior cingulate gyri may explain the attention deficit commonly experienced by patients with TBI.

Doshi and colleagues[43] expanded the scope of TBI research using ASL to include emergency room patients with mTBI in the early stages, with time delay to scan ranging between 3 hours and 10 days. Using ASL and susceptibility weighted imaging, they found increased rCBF in the caudate, putamen, and ventral pallidum of the subjects with mTBI. Although there is a wide distribution of delayed scan times among subjects, the increase in rCBF contrasts sharply with the decreased CBF found in previous studies, which the investigators attribute to the early versus chronic phases of TBI injury and to the mild versus severe degrees of injuries.

In a recent study, MR imaging was performed on both contact sports athletes (ie, football players) and non–contact sports athletes (ie, volleyball players).[44] There was no difference in the volumes of the cortex, white matter, basal ganglia, thalami, or hippocampi between the two groups.[44] However, the football players had significantly lower CBV than the volleyball players in the hippocampi and thalami, which suggests that CBV may be a more sensitive metric for detecting TBI (Fig. 5).[44]

Challenges of Arterial Spin Labeling MR Imaging in Acute Traumatic Brain Injury

One technical challenge of applying ASL to TBI imaging lies in its inherently low signal/noise ratio (SNR) and temporal resolution.[45] Because the signal from labeled inflow water protons constitutes only 0.5% to 1.5% of the total tissue signal, ASL is an inherently low-SNR technique. SNR can be improved by averaging over repeated acquisitions, increasing magnetic field strength, reducing patient movement, and using fast-imaging techniques such as echo-planar imaging (EPI) and phase-array receiver coils for parallel imaging. However, EPI can suffer from image distortion in regions with high magnetic susceptibilities. Newer pulse sequences, such as turbo-ASL[46] and single-shot ASL,[47] can shorten acquisition times, but the interpretation of the signal is more complicated.

Apparent discrepancies between results published by different research groups in terms of the changes of ASL signals and CBF associated with TBI were highlighted earlier. CBF seems to increase in certain brain regions; for example, the caudate and putamen in the acute phase immediately after impact.[43] It has been shown at the cellular level that cortical impact causes neuronal loss, axonal injury, blood-brain barrier (BBB) disruption, and microscopic hemorrhage between days 1 and 28 post-TBI.[48] The acute CBF change may reflect the brain's autoregulatory mechanism to maintain constant perfusion by a compensatory increase in blood flow. During the chronic phase of moderate to severe TBI, there is a global decline in perfusion, especially in thalami and posterior cingulate gyri, accompanied by volume loss in the lesions.[42]

Additional research is needed to elucidate the physiologic transition between the early and chronic phases in mTBI and severe TBI. In addition, the exact mechanism underlying cognitive impairment from TBI is yet to be discovered.[38] Clearly ASL alone cannot capture the complex physiologic changes in an injured brain along time and space axes; the armamentarium of neuroimaging techniques reviewed thus far must be used together to collect information on the white and gray matter changes, CBF/CBV, BBB permeability, microvascular capacity, and oxygen delivery and metabolism rates after an injury occurs, thereby constructing a comprehensive and consistent framework to describe the physiologic basis of TBI in vivo.

STABLE XENON PERFUSION COMPUTED TOMOGRAPHY
Introduction

Another form of PCT imaging is performed by inhalation of stable xenon gas instead of injecting iodinated contrast. In xenon PCT, images are acquired during both a wash-in phase and a wash-out phase of the xenon gas. One protocol that has been studied in multiple trials includes a protocol of 13 to 17 minutes consisting of 4 axial slices each measuring 5 mm thick with 20 mm of spacing between slices.[49–51]

Xenon Computed Tomography Imaging Applied to Acute Traumatic Brain Injury

In one study of 90 patients with TBI, Xe-CT performed 1 to 3 days post-TBI was correlated with outcomes.[52] MTT was measured with a region of interest including the average of the right and left hemispheres measured at the level of the basal ganglia.[52] Discriminate analysis based on a cutoff MTT value of 6.85 seconds predicted good outcomes (good recovery and moderate disability) and bad outcomes (severe disability, vegetative state, and death) with an accuracy of 70.6%.[52]

In another study, stable Xe-CT imaging was used within 12 hours of severe TBI to determine whether neurologic outcome measured by Glasgow Outcome Scale (GOS) could be predicted by early CBF.[51] Xe-CT was able to distinguish GOS 1 to 2 (dead or vegetative state) from GOS 3 to 5 (severely disabled to good recovery) with a receiver operating characteristic curve area under the curve of 0.92 at 6 hours and 0.77 at 12 hours.[51] This finding emphasizes the importance of early perfusion imaging after TBI.

Challenges of Stable Xenon Computed Tomography Imaging in Acute Traumatic Brain Injury

The most significant challenge in recent years is that stable xenon of medical quality is largely unavailable in the United States. For this reason, clinical use and research of Xe-CT is on hold at this time.

FUTURE PERFUSION RESEARCH

Neuroprotective strategies have resulted in positive outcomes in animal research. However, such preclinical successes have failed to translate into improved clinical outcomes in clinical TBI trials.[53–56] One possible explanation for this is that there is more heterogeneity in TBI in clinical settings compared with consistent models in animal research.[51,53,57] The importance of early perfusion changes has been recognized in TBI for its prognostic value.[23,51] Thus, one area of further research should be in early post-TBI perfusion changes.

The benefits of early perfusion are well known and it is commonly used in seizure localization through the use of technetium-99m (Tc-99m) HMPAO. Tc99m HMPAO is taken up rapidly within the brain (30–60 seconds) and its long half-life allows high-quality scanning up to 4 hours after the injection. The distribution of the tracer at the time of the imaging provides a snapshot of the blood flow at the moment of tracer injection. Despite the known utility of performing ictal SPECT imaging with Tc-99m HMPAO for seizure localization,[58] a recent systematic review SPECT imaging at TBI revealed that 19 longitudinal and 52 cross-sectional studies only found a single study that was performed within 12 hours of the TBI.[59,60] This study showed hypoperfusion after TBI and found that the hypoperfusion correlated with amnesia.[60]

An ongoing Department of Defense–funded TBI study is investigating early perfusion changes in the acute phase of TBI.[61] An animal model with precision cortical impact is being followed by Tc-99m HMPAO tracer administration with subsequent SPECT-CT imaging within the half-life of the tracer. The experimental design reflects the realistic scenario of brain injury sustained by a soldier in combat who receives the radiopharmaceutical injection and subsequent SPECT-CT imaging within a few hours. In our TBI animal experiments, decreased perfusion was seen at the cortical impact site (Fig. 6), consistent with hypoperfusion observed by other research groups.[61] A limitation of this technique is the poor spatial resolution of SPECT-CT. Future experiments will soon be conducted with high-spatial-resolution collimators.

The considerable heterogeneity in TBI poses a challenge in identifying an effective treatment at an individual level[62]; however, perfusion imaging creates new opportunities for detection of injuries that might otherwise go unnoticed with conventional imaging. Through perfusion imaging, more specific diagnoses can be made and coupled with more specific treatments. Future research may involve building normal age-stratified perfusion imaging scans. With a normative database, computer-aided diagnosis and machine learning (ML) could be performed, yielding a more refined diagnosis through etiologic, symptom-based, or prognostic classifications of TBI.[63–66] ML refers to the process of training a computer algorithm to "learn" from past experience where perfusion parameters (eg, CBV values) are matched to particular outcomes (eg, GOS). An integrated approach that combines optimal structural

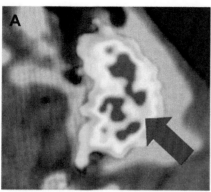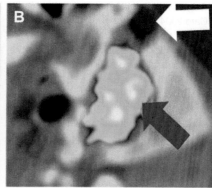

Fig. 6. Two Tc-99m-HMPAO images of molecular neuroimaging of cerebral blood flow abnormalities caused by TBI in a swine model (*Sus scrofa*). Control (*A*) shows normal perfusion (*red arrow*). The 1-hour post-TBI image (*B*) shows the craniectomy site (*white arrow*) at the top of the image with hypoperfusion seen in the underlying brain (*red arrow*).

imaging, perfusion imaging, and clinical parameters may direct future treatment directions.

SUMMARY

TBI is a significant problem worldwide and neuroimaging plays a critical role in diagnosis and management. In this article, CT bolus perfusion, MR imaging bolus perfusion, MR imaging ASL perfusion, and Xe-CT are reviewed with a focus on their application in TBI. Future research directions are also discussed.

REFERENCES

1. Faul M, National Center for Injury Prevention and Control (U.S.). Traumatic brain injury in the United States: emergency department visits, hospitalizations, and deaths, 2002-2006. Available at: http://purl.fdlp.gov/GPO/gpo41911. Accessed April 25, 2017.
2. Marin JR, Weaver MD, Yealy DM, et al. Trends in visits for traumatic brain injury to emergency departments in the United States. JAMA 2014;311(18):1917–9.
3. Centers for Disease Control and Prevention. Nonfatal traumatic brain injuries related to sports and recreation activities among persons aged </=19 years–United States, 2001-2009. MMWR Morb Mortal Wkly Rep 2011;60(39):1337–42.
4. Corrigan JD, Selassie AW, Orman JA. The epidemiology of traumatic brain injury. J Head Trauma Rehabil 2010;25(2):72–80.
5. Bass E, Golding H, United States. Congressional Budget Office. The Veterans Health Administration's treatment of PTSD and traumatic brain injury among recent combat veterans. A CBO study. Washington, DC: United States Publishing Office; 2012. Available at: http://purl.fdlp.gov/GPO/gpo18872. Accessed April 25, 2017.
6. Shetty VS, Reis MN, Aulino JM, et al. ACR appropriateness criteria head trauma. J Am Coll Radiol 2016; 13(6):668–79.
7. Servadei F, Nasi MT, Giuliani G, et al. CT prognostic factors in acute subdural haematomas: the value of the 'worst' CT scan. Br J Neurosurg 2000;14(2):110–6.
8. Celli P, Fruin A, Cervoni L. Severe head trauma. Review of the factors influencing the prognosis. Minerva Chir 1997;52(12):1467–80.
9. Lev MH, Segal AZ, Farkas J, et al. Utility of perfusion-weighted CT imaging in acute middle cerebral artery stroke treated with intra-arterial thrombolysis: prediction of final infarct volume and clinical outcome. Stroke 2001;32(9):2021–8.
10. Wintermark M, Reichhart M, Thiran JP, et al. Prognostic accuracy of cerebral blood flow measurement by perfusion computed tomography, at the time of emergency room admission, in acute stroke patients. Ann Neurol 2002;51(4):417–32.
11. Wintermark M, Reichhart M, Cuisenaire O, et al. Comparison of admission perfusion computed tomography and qualitative diffusion- and perfusion-weighted magnetic resonance imaging in acute stroke patients. Stroke 2002;33(8):2025–31.
12. Wintermark M, Maeder P, Thiran JP, et al. Quantitative assessment of regional cerebral blood flows by perfusion CT studies at low injection rates: a critical review of the underlying theoretical models. Eur Radiol 2001;11(7):1220–30.
13. Garnett MR, Blamire AM, Corkill RG, et al. Abnormal cerebral blood volume in regions of contused and normal appearing brain following traumatic brain injury using perfusion magnetic resonance imaging. J Neurotrauma 2001;18(6):585–93.
14. Menon DK. Brain ischaemia after traumatic brain injury: lessons from 15O2 positron emission tomography. Curr Opin Crit Care 2006;12(2):85–9.

15. Coles JP. Regional ischemia after head injury. Curr Opin Crit Care 2004;10(2):120–5.

16. Cunningham AS, Salvador R, Coles JP, et al. Physiological thresholds for irreversible tissue damage in contusional regions following traumatic brain injury. Brain 2005;128(Pt 8):1931–42.

17. Wintermark M, Thiran JP, Maeder P, et al. Simultaneous measurement of regional cerebral blood flow by perfusion CT and stable xenon CT: a validation study. AJNR Am J Neuroradiol 2001;22(5):905–14.

18. Axel L. Cerebral blood flow determination by rapid-sequence computed tomography: theoretical analysis. Radiology 1980;137(3):679–86.

19. Axel L. A method of calculating brain blood flow with a CT dynamic scanner. Adv Neurol 1981;30:67–71.

20. Axel L. Tissue mean transit time from dynamic computed tomography by a simple deconvolution technique. Invest Radiol 1983;18(1):94–9.

21. Bivard A, Levi C, Spratt N, et al. Perfusion CT in acute stroke: a comprehensive analysis of infarct and penumbra. Radiology 2013;267(2):543–50.

22. Latchaw RE, Yonas H, Hunter GJ, et al. Guidelines and recommendations for perfusion imaging in cerebral ischemia: a scientific statement for healthcare professionals by the writing group on perfusion imaging, from the Council on Cardiovascular Radiology of the American Heart Association. Stroke 2003;34(4):1084–104.

23. Wintermark M, van Melle G, Schnyder P, et al. Admission perfusion CT: prognostic value in patients with severe head trauma. Radiology 2004;232(1):211–20.

24. Metting Z, Rodiger LA, de Jong BM, et al. Acute cerebral perfusion CT abnormalities associated with posttraumatic amnesia in mild head injury. J Neurotrauma 2010;27(12):2183–9.

25. Bendinelli C, Bivard A, Nebauer S, et al. Brain CT perfusion provides additional useful information in severe traumatic brain injury. Injury 2013;44(9):1208–12.

26. Soustiel JF, Mahamid E, Goldsher D, et al. Perfusion-CT for early assessment of traumatic cerebral contusions. Neuroradiology 2008;50(2):189–96.

27. Wintermark M, Maeder P, Verdun FR, et al. Using 80 kVp versus 120 kVp in perfusion CT measurement of regional cerebral blood flow. AJNR Am J Neuroradiol 2000;21(10):1881–4.

28. McGehee BE, Pollock JM, Maldjian JA. Brain perfusion imaging: how does it work and what should I use? J Magn Reson Imaging 2012;36(6):1257–72.

29. Liu W, Wang B, Wolfowitz R, et al. Perfusion deficits in patients with mild traumatic brain injury characterized by dynamic susceptibility contrast MRI. NMR Biomed 2013;26(6):651–63.

30. Williams DS, Detre JA, Leigh JS, et al. Magnetic resonance imaging of perfusion using spin inversion of arterial water. Proc Natl Acad Sci U S A 1992;89(1):212–6.

31. Deibler AR, Pollock JM, Kraft RA, et al. Arterial spin-labeling in routine clinical practice, part 1: technique and artifacts. AJNR Am J Neuroradiol 2008;29(7):1228–34.

32. Deibler AR, Pollock JM, Kraft RA, et al. Arterial spin-labeling in routine clinical practice, part 2: hypoperfusion patterns. AJNR Am J Neuroradiol 2008;29(7):1235–41.

33. Deibler AR, Pollock JM, Kraft RA, et al. Arterial spin-labeling in routine clinical practice, part 3: hyperperfusion patterns. AJNR Am J Neuroradiol 2008;29(8):1428–35.

34. Johnson NA, Jahng GH, Weiner MW, et al. Pattern of cerebral hypoperfusion in Alzheimer disease and mild cognitive impairment measured with arterial spin-labeling MR imaging: initial experience. Radiology 2005;234(3):851–9.

35. Bokkers RP, Bremmer JP, van Berckel BN, et al. Arterial spin labeling perfusion MRI at multiple delay times: a correlative study with H(2)(15)O positron emission tomography in patients with symptomatic carotid artery occlusion. J Cereb Blood Flow Metab 2010;30(1):222–9.

36. Zaharchuk G, Do HM, Marks MP, et al. Arterial spin-labeling MRI can identify the presence and intensity of collateral perfusion in patients with moyamoya disease. Stroke 2011;42(9):2485–91.

37. Gevers S, van Osch MJ, Bokkers RP, et al. Intra- and multicenter reproducibility of pulsed, continuous and pseudo-continuous arterial spin labeling methods for measuring cerebral perfusion. J Cereb Blood Flow Metab 2011;31(8):1706–15.

38. Wang Y, West JD, Bailey JN, et al. Decreased cerebral blood flow in chronic pediatric mild TBI: an MRI perfusion study. Dev Neuropsychol 2015;40(1):40–4.

39. Petcharunpaisan S, Ramalho J, Castillo M. Arterial spin labeling in neuroimaging. World J Radiol 2010;2(10):384–98.

40. Kochanek PM, Hendrich KS, Dixon CE, et al. Cerebral blood flow at one year after controlled cortical impact in rats: assessment by magnetic resonance imaging. J Neurotrauma 2002;19(9):1029–37.

41. Ge Y, Patel MB, Chen Q, et al. Assessment of thalamic perfusion in patients with mild traumatic brain injury by true FISP arterial spin labelling MR imaging at 3T. Brain Inj 2009;23(7):666–74.

42. Kim J, Whyte J, Patel S, et al. Resting cerebral blood flow alterations in chronic traumatic brain injury: an arterial spin labeling perfusion FMRI study. J Neurotrauma 2010;27(8):1399–411.

43. Doshi H, Wiseman N, Liu J, et al. Cerebral hemodynamic changes of mild traumatic brain injury at the acute stage. PLoS One 2015;10(2):e0118061.

44. Zeineh M, Douglas DB, Parekh M, et al. Alteration of cerebral blood flow in contact-sport athletes. American Society of Neuroradiology Annual Conference. Chicago, April 20-25, 2015.

45. Andre JB. Arterial spin labeling magnetic resonance perfusion for traumatic brain injury: technical challenges and potentials. Top Magn Reson Imaging 2015;24(5):275–87.

46. Wong EC, Cronin M, Wu WC, et al. Velocity-selective arterial spin labeling. Magn Reson Med 2006;55(6): 1334–41.

47. Duyn JH, Tan CX, van Gelderen P, et al. High-sensitivity single-shot perfusion-weighted fMRI. Magn Reson Med 2001;46(1):88–94.

48. Chen S, Pickard JD, Harris NG. Time course of cellular pathology after controlled cortical impact injury. Exp Neurol 2003;182(1):87–102.

49. Hlatky R, Contant CF, Diaz-Marchan P, et al. Significance of a reduced cerebral blood flow during the first 12 hours after traumatic brain injury. Neurocrit Care 2004;1(1):69–83.

50. Yonas H, Darby JM, Marks EC, et al. CBF measured by Xe-CT: approach to analysis and normal values. J Cereb Blood flow Metab 1991;11(5):716–25.

51. Kaloostian P, Robertson C, Gopinath SP, et al. Outcome prediction within twelve hours after severe traumatic brain injury by quantitative cerebral blood flow. J Neurotrauma 2012;29(5):727–34.

52. Honda M, Ichibayashi R, Yokomuro H, et al. Early cerebral circulation disturbance in patients suffering from severe traumatic brain injury (TBI): a xenon CT and perfusion CT study. Neurol Med Chir (Tokyo) 2016;56(8):501–9.

53. Jain KK. Neuroprotection in traumatic brain injury. Drug Discov Today 2008;13(23–24):1082–9.

54. Bullock MR, Lyeth BG, Muizelaar JP. Current status of neuroprotection trials for traumatic brain injury: lessons from animal models and clinical studies. Neurosurgery 1999;45(2):207–17 [discussion: 217–20].

55. Narayan RK, Michel ME, Ansell B, et al. Clinical trials in head injury. J Neurotrauma 2002;19(5):503–57.

56. Tolias CM, Bullock MR. Critical appraisal of neuroprotection trials in head injury: what have we learned? NeuroRx 2004;1(1):71–9.

57. Loane DJ, Faden AI. Neuroprotection for traumatic brain injury: translational challenges and emerging therapeutic strategies. Trends Pharmacol Sci 2010; 31(12):596–604.

58. Lapalme-Remis S, Cascino GD. Imaging for adults with seizures and epilepsy. Continuum (Minneap Minn) 2016;22(5, Neuroimaging):1451–79.

59. Raji CA, Tarzwell R, Pavel D, et al. Clinical utility of SPECT neuroimaging in the diagnosis and treatment of traumatic brain injury: a systematic review. PLoS One 2014;9(3):e91088.

60. Lorberboym M, Lampl Y, Gerzon I, et al. Brain SPECT evaluation of amnestic ED patients after mild head trauma. Am J Emerg Med 2002;20(4): 310–3.

61. Douglas DB, Douglas JM, Zhao JW. A pilot study of molecular neuroimaging of cerebral blood flow abnormalities due to traumatic brain injury (TBI) in swine model. Travis Air Force Base (CA): David Grant Medical Center; 2015.

62. Saatman KE, Duhaime AC, Bullock R, et al. Classification of traumatic brain injury for targeted therapies. J Neurotrauma 2008;25(7):719–38.

63. Mourao-Miranda J, Bokde AL, Born C, et al. Classifying brain states and determining the discriminating activation patterns: support vector machine on functional MRI data. Neuroimage 2005;28(4): 980–95.

64. De Martino F, Valente G, Staeren N, et al. Combining multivariate voxel selection and support vector machines for mapping and classification of fMRI spatial patterns. Neuroimage 2008;43(1):44–58.

65. Friston KJ. Modalities, modes, and models in functional neuroimaging. Science 2009;326(5951): 399–403.

66. Burges JC. A tutorial on support vector machines for pattern recognition. Data Min Knowl Discov 1998;2: 121–67.

PET and Single-Photon Emission Computed Tomography in Brain Concussion

Cyrus A. Raji, MD, PhD[a],
Theodore A. Henderson, MD, PhD[b],*

KEYWORDS

- Concussion ● Mild traumatic brain injury ● PET ● SPECT ● TBI ● CTE

KEY POINTS

- Neuronuclear procedures use radiopharmaceuticals, which produce gamma radiation; the distribution of gamma radiation is captured by gamma cameras and processed for 3-dimensional distribution and radiopharmaceutical density.
- Neuronuclear procedures (PET, single-photon emission computed tomography [SPECT] scan) provide information about the functional activity within different parts of the brain.
- The risk of cancer or radiation injury associated with neuronuclear imaging with a radiation dose of 0.8 rem or less remains hypothetical.
- PET with fludeoxyglucose F 18 neuroimaging studies of mild traumatic brain injury (mTBI) or concussion have been limited, with a total of less than 100 subjects.
- SPECT studies of TBI encompass thousands of subjects. Given the shortcomings of post-processing metrics in fMRI and the recent advances in SPECT quantitative analysis, SPECT offers a promising opportunity to assess TBI, even mTBI, and provide both screening and post-injury monitoring quantitative data.

INTRODUCTION

Concussion is now recognized to be a form of mild traumatic brain injury (mTBI). Until recently, concussion was thought to be inconsequential and spontaneously resolving.[1] Currently, an explosion of epidemiologic, neurologic, and pathologic studies is beginning to reveal the subacute, chronic, and long-term consequences of concussion. Research has demonstrated that even single concussions can have lasting effects and multiple subconcussive impacts can have an accumulative effect, leading to significant pathologic changes.[1,2] The costs of concussion and TBI were estimated in 2010 at $11.5 billion in direct medical costs and $64.8 billion in lost wages and productivity.[3]

Disclosures: Dr C.A. Raji received consulting fees from the Change Your Brain Change Your Life Foundation and Brainreader ApS. T.A. Henderson is the president and principal owner of The Synaptic Space, a neuroimaging consulting firm. He is owner of Neuro-Luminance Corporation, a medical service company. He is also president and principal owner of Dr. Theodore Henderson, Inc, a medical service company. He is also Vice-President of the Neuro-Laser Foundation, a non-profit organization. Currently, he serves as president of the International Society of Applied Neuroimaging.
[a] Department of Radiology and Biomedical Imaging, University of California, San Francisco, UCSF China Basin, 185 Berry Street, Suite 350, San Francisco, CA 94158, USA; [b] The Synaptic Space Inc, Neuro-Laser Foundation, Neuro-Luminance Brain Health Centers Inc, Dr. Theodore Henderson Inc, 3979 East Arapahoe Road, Suite 200, Centennial, CO 80122, USA
* Corresponding author.
E-mail address: thesynapticspace7@gmail.com

Neuroimag Clin N Am 28 (2018) 67–82
https://doi.org/10.1016/j.nic.2017.09.003

The increased vulnerability of certain populations—women, the elderly, and the young—is emerging. For example, the incidence of concussion among women playing a given sport is 1.4 to 3.7 times greater than for men playing the same sport, including those less violent sports.[4,5] The elderly are considerably more like to be admitted to hospital after a TBI of any severity.[6] Falls represent the largest cause of TBI in the elderly, followed by motor vehicle accidents. Despite having less severe injuries in general, the elderly have higher mortality and worse functional outcomes.[7–11] The elderly have a considerably higher incidence of subdural hematoma after TBI of any severity, possibly owing to atrophy and the concomitant strain on the dural vessels, as well as the extensive use of aspirin and anticoagulant therapy.[12]

At the opposite end of the age spectrum, the brain of youth is more vulnerable to injury owing to the incomplete myelination of large portions of the cerebral cortex. This condition results in greater friability, which increases with decreasing age. In the United States, children and adolescents are most likely to experience concussion in sports and recreation. It should be noted that 70% of all US football players are under age 14.[13] A helmet sensor study of 50 child football players, ages 9 to 12, revealed more than 11,900 helmet impacts in 1 season.[13] Urban and colleagues[14] reported there were 16,500 impacts among 40 high school football players in 1 season. The current focus on the risks of chronic traumatic encephalopathy (CTE) for professional football players ignores the impact and long-term risk of childhood concussions in the evolution of CTE.[15–17] For example, former NFL player Tyler Sash died at age 27 and donated his brain to study CTE. According to a 2016 *New York Times* article, his brain showed extensive accumulation of the abnormal tau protein involved in CTE, similar to a large proportion of professional football players examined to date.[18] So Tyler, only 9 years out of high school, already had CTE. His brain injuries likely began when he was a pee-wee football player, extended through high school, college, and his very short professional career. A recent study showed 21% of children with concussion have persistent symptoms.[19] Stamm and colleagues[20] found that football players who started tackle football before age 12 had greater cognitive impairment as they age.

In our opinion, there is an urgent need to be able to distinguish those patients with concussion or mTBI who are at risk for persistent postconcussive symptoms and tauopathy. This information will be critical in return-to-play decisions at any age. Moreover, prioritizing treatment and advising future sports and recreational behaviors for those at risk of persistent pathologic changes will be critical public health concerns. The glaring deficit in the diagnosis and treatment of concussion and mTBI has been the absence of a method of accurately imaging the injury.

In this article, the potential strengths of PET and single-photon emission computed tomography (SPECT) neuroimaging compared with other forms of neuroimaging are illustrated. **Fig. 1** shows example brain SPECT and PET scans. These nuclear medicine procedures often are avoided out of concern for radiation exposure. Consequently, the radiation risk issues of SPECT and PET scans are initially reviewed. The current state-of-the-art literature for both SPECT and PET imaging in TBI, with a particular focus on mTBI, is presented.

RADIATION RISK

An oft-cited criticism against neuronuclear imaging techniques, whether it is SPECT perfusion neuroimaging or PET metabolic imaging, is the associated risk of radiation exposure. A PET scan on average carries a 700 mRems exposure,[21] and a computed tomography (CT) scan of the head can lead to an exposure of 800 to 900 mRems,[21] depending on the imaging protocol. A perfusion SPECT scan of the brain carries 640 mRems of exposure.[21] This amount is approximately 2 times the range of typical background exposure from the natural environment and modern technology, such as smoke detectors, televisions, computers, and air travel.[22] The natural background radiation exposure in the United States is 293 mRems in coastal areas and 387 mRems in the mountainous areas of Colorado.[22] **Table 1** displays these comparisons in units of mSv and Rems.

The theoretic debate in the field of radiation exposure risk is whether or not there is a linear no-threshold model or a threshold model for risk associated with radiation exposure. The proponents of the linear no-threshold model hold that all radiation is potentially harmful, as summarized by Howe and McLaughlin[23] and the BEIR V report.[24] The studies often cited as supporting the linear no-threshold model, in fact, on close examination do not support the linear model. In particular, Howe and McLaughlin[23] report increased cancer rate among women exposed to chest fluoroscopy, but these data clearly demonstrate a decreased risk at doses below 2 rem.[25] Likewise, a study by the International Agency for Research on Cancer[26] involving 95,673 subjects demonstrated a negative correlation between low-level radiation exposure and the risk of solid tumors. In addition, the risk of leukemias in this

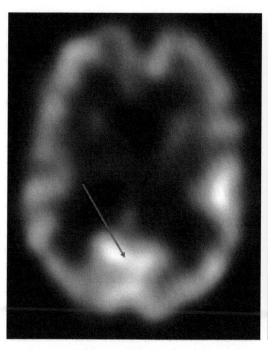

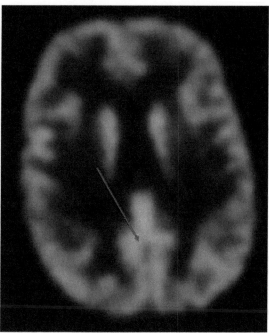

BRAIN SPECT SCAN

BRAIN PET SCAN

Fig. 1. Two axial images, one of a brain single-photon emission computed tomography (SPECT) scan and one of a brain PET scan. The *arrows* point to the posterior cingulate gyrus on both scans, highlighting the healthy perfusion on brain SPECT and the normal fluorodeoxyglucose metabolism on PET imaging.

Table 1
Radiation exposures of common diagnostic procedures relative to background exposures

Source	mSv	Rems
Background radiation	2.93	0.293
Background radiation (Denver)	3.87	0.387
Chest radiograph	0.09	.009
Airport x-ray scanner	0.003	0.0003
Jet flight (8 h)	0.04	0.004
Lumbar spine radiograph series	0.13	0.013
Head computed tomography scan	9.13	0.913
Interventional fluoroscopy (5 min)	7.00	0.7
SPECT (adult)	6.80	0.68
SPECT (child)	2.20	0.22
PET (adult)	7.03	0.703

Abbreviation: SPECT, single-photon emission computed tomography.

Data from RADAR Home. Available at: http://www. doseinfo-radar.com/. Accessed January 31, 2017; and United States Environmental Protection Agency. Radiation protection: calculate your radiation dose website. Available at: https://www.epa.gov/radiation/calculate-your-radiation-dose. Accessed January 31, 2017.

large, epidemiologic study was increased only at doses exceeding 4 rem.[26]

The recent BEIR VII report in 2006 took the position that there is no lower limit to the cancer risk associated with radiation exposure.[24] The conclusions of the BEIR committee, based on extrapolation of data from Hiroshima survivors, estimate a 1% increase in the rate of cancer with exposure to 100 mSv. Extending this logic from high-dose exposure to doses as low as 10 mSv associated with neuronuclear imaging procedures yields a risk of 1 in 1000 for increased cancer. However, experts assert that it is not clear that an increased rate of cancer could be detected at these low radiation exposure levels.[27–32] Statistically, it is unlikely we can detect a one-tenth of 1% increase in cancer rate when roughly 1,530,000 cases of cancer occur each year in the United States.[25,32] However, there is extensive evidence against long-term risk associated with a low level of radiation exposure.[31,32] For example, Saenger and colleagues[30] reported on the long-term follow-up of 18,379 patients treated with I-131 for hyperthyroidism with an average dose of 10 rem to bone marrow (range, 7–15 rem), compared with nonirradiated subjects, and found no increased rate of leukemia. Similarly, Ron and Modan[31] reported a sample of 11,000 patients under the age of 15 years treated with radiation for tinea capitis with an average dose of 9.3 rem (range, 4.5–50). Compared with 16,000 controls at 22 years of follow-up, there was no difference in rate of leukemia. In summary, the risk of cancer or radiation injury associated with SPECT scans with a radiation dose of only 0.68 rem or PET scans at a radiation dose of 0.70 rem remains hypothetical, because there are no published data demonstrating an actual quantitative increase in cancer rates associated with neuronuclear scans. But, what is the overall risk of undergoing an SPECT scan or a PET scan? A leading authority on the subject of medical radiation exposure, Dr Michael Devous, has stated in several settings,[33,34] "that there are no data that have ever demonstrated any harm to humans by radiation exposures at diagnostic imaging levels (emphasis added). In fact, current data support the presence of radiation hormesis; that low levels of radiation exposure induce beneficial effects of cellular repair and immune system enhancement. Therefore, it should be concluded that neither SPECT nor PET brain imaging procedures are associated with any particular risk over activities of daily living and certainly should not be considered to be any more risky than MRI or any of its associated functional imaging derivatives."

The Health Physics Society in their 2004 and 2009 position papers[27] states, "the Health Physics Society recommends against quantitative estimation of health risks below an individual dose of 5 rem in 1 year or a lifetime dose of 10 rem…There is substantial and convincing scientific evidence for health risks at high-dose exposure. However, below 5 to 10 rem (which includes occupational and environmental exposures) risks of health effects are too small to be observed or are nonexistent."

Similarly, the American Nuclear Society in its 2001 position paper[28] states, "there is insufficient scientific evidence to support the use of the Linear No Threshold Hypothesis (LNTH) in the projection of effects of low-level radiation."

THE PHYSICS OF SINGLE-PHOTON EMISSION COMPUTED TOMOGRAPHY

SPECT scanning provides 3-dimensional (3-D) information about the distribution of a radiopharmaceutical within a patient. SPECT radiopharmaceuticals generally emit gamma rays and multiple radionuclides with differing gamma photon energies are used. The most common radionuclides (with corresponding gamma photon energies) are technetium-99m (140 keV), thallium-201 (72 keV), iodine-123 (159 keV), iodine-125 (35 keV), and xenon-133 (81 keV). The most commonly used radiopharmaceuticals for the study of the brain are xenon-133, 99mTc-hexamethylpropylene amine oxime (HMPAO), Tc99m-ethylcysteinate dimer for perfusion imaging, and DatScan for dopamine transporter imaging. Other radiopharmaceuticals used in research allow localization of different receptors (eg, serotonin, benzodiazepine, opiate).

SPECT imaging is based on triangulating on the site of the radiopharmaceutical that is directly releasing a photon. Thus, the resolution is potentially to a point source of photons. The resolution limits of SPECT scans stem from the physical collimation and the relative size of photodetectors. SPECT scanning combines CT methods with scintigraphy. A typical SPECT instrument in use for the past 20 years used 2 or more scintillation cameras or heads that rotate about the patient. Older SPECT instruments used a single camera or head and yielded images of considerably lower resolution. Essentially, each head consists of a collimator in front of a sodium iodide scintillation crystal, which in turn is in front of a photomultiplier array. The sodium iodide crystal converts a gamma photon strike into a visible light emission. The photomultiplier array, in turn, amplifies the light emission. A position logic circuit, referred to as an Anger circuit, determines the relative position of the gamma photon strikes on the crystal and a 2-dimensional image of the 3-D distribution of radioactivity is formed.

Until recently, the collimation system has depended on lead collimators, which eliminate as much as 60% of the emitted photons. Parallel hole collimators have classically been used and are superior for quantitative analysis. Converging or fan beam collimators increase photon passage by 150% to 200%, but yield a smaller field of view. Although this stringent collimation largely eliminates scatter and increases spatial resolution, it has necessitated larger radiopharmaceutical doses and longer scan times to achieve adequate counts. Recently, a technological advancement of significance is the ongoing development by Project ProSPECTus of a modern Compton Camera system.[35] The essentials of the design are the alignment of 2 parallel detectors. The first registers in position of the incident gamma radiation, while inducing Compton scatter. The second detector registers the position of the scattered photon. The measurements of the position and energy of the photon at both detectors is used to calculate the angle and position of the source of the gamma photon.[35] This new camera technology would be at least 100 times more sensitive than the current SPECT cameras, with dramatically superior spatial resolutions of 2 to 3 mm. The technology also is compatible with MR imaging and could potentially be retrofitted to current MR imaging machines.

Perhaps the most important recent advance in SPECT imaging is the cadmium–zinc–telluride (CZT) detector. The CZT detector functions as a semiconductor with direct conversion of gamma radiation to an electric signal. The CZT detector eliminates the need for photomultipliers. Also, low-energy collimators are replaced with pinhole collimators with better energy resolution. This mechanism results in better spatial resolution and sensitivity, which means a lower administered dose of radiopharmaceuticals and/or shorter acquisition times. CZT detectors increase the count sensitivity by about 3-fold[36] and have an intrinsic spatial resolution of 2.5 mm. The full width half-maximum is 1.73 to 3.88 mm compared with a full width half-maximum of 8.17 to 12.63 mm with a sodium iodide photomultiplier system.[37]

The relatively low energy of gamma emitters used in SPECT radiopharmaceuticals results in greater attenuation and Compton scatter compared with the 511 keV gamma photons used in PET imaging. For example, it is estimated that approximately 50% of Tc-99m photons are lost in 4.5 cm of water or soft tissue. Attenuation correction algorithms applied during image processing can correct for this and the availability of SPECT/CT cameras allow for more accurate CT-based attenuation correction. Photons can alter their trajectory through tissue owing to Compton interactions. The scattered photons have reduced energy and can be detected and excluded from the final image. This maneuver is typically performed after photomultiplication using a pulse height analyzer with a narrow energy window centered on the keV of the radionuclide of interest.

The most elementary of SPECT reconstruction methods is filtered backprojection. This method, in simple terms, uses the projection ray of photons that sum to yield a single point in the 2-dimensional representation of the 3-D distribution of radioactivity and projects it back on itself and also at multiples of 45° off parallel. This method increases relative counts in the image of structures with high radioactivity counts, but also creates a star-shaped blurring. The blurring effect is corrected using a filter, often a variable ramp filter. Filtered backprojection can amplify statistical noise. An alternate method is iterative reconstruction, which essentially uses comparisons of multiple iterations of the reconstruction to a template generated from the original data. With thousands of iterations, the template is a progressively more accurate representation of the actual distribution of radionuclide. A further refinement of iterative reconstruction is ordered sets expectation maximization. This method uses subsets of the projection data to perform iterative reconstruction toward expectation maximization. The solution of each subset was used as a starting point for the analysis of the next subset.

Quantitative analysis of image data yields a much greater understanding of disease processes compared with visual read alone. An early approach was region of interest (ROI) analysis, wherein regions were defined, often by hand drawing of the boundaries in 2-dimensional slices of the scan, and compared across conditions. If the scans of multiple subjects can be normalized spatially to a 3-D template of the human brain, then the voxels within a predetermined 3-D region can be analyzed. Taking this a step further, statistical comparison at each voxel can be conducted between subjects or groups of subjects in a process known as statistical parametric analysis. Another method of (semi)quantitative analysis of functional neuroimaging depends on the standardized uptake value (SUV). The SUV is a ratio of the tissue concentration of a tracer compared with a reference region, often the entire structure, followed by normalization for dose, patient volume, and radionuclide decay. Theoretically, SUV reduces variance from differences in patient size and radiopharmaceutical dose. Nevertheless, these sources of variance are not completely overcome. Standardization across scanners is problematic and instrument-specific SUV protocols yield superior results. These topics are reviewed in detail elsewhere.[38,39]

SPECT scanning is the most enduring and the most widely available technology for measuring brain function.[33,34,40–42] SPECT facilities outnumber PET facilities 12-fold.[34,42] Using currently available radiopharmaceuticals, perfusion SPECT scanning accurately represents regional cerebral blood flow.[43,44] Additional tracers have become available to measure receptor density and dopamine transporter site density. Although these tracers provide valuable information about certain neuronal systems, this article focuses on regional cerebral blood flow as a measure of brain function in health and in traumatic brain injury (TBI).

Regional cerebral blood flow is a valid marker for neuronal activity over most of the physiologic range of cerebral blood flow. This is because, under most neurophysiologic circumstances, the regional cerebral blood flow is tightly coupled to neuronal metabolism. This principle underlies SPECT perfusion imaging and functional MR imaging. One importance difference between functional MR imaging and SPECT scanning is that functional MR imaging has a much smaller relative signal change, resulting in the need for extensive postprocessing manipulation. This postprocessing rendering has recently been shown to have potential errors in the underlying statistical models, potentially invalidating numerous previously published functional MR imaging studies.[45] SPECT perfusion was first measured with xenon (133Xe), an inert gas that precisely quantifies cerebral blood flow. Commonly used radiopharmaceuticals currently include HMPAO, 99mTc- ethylcysteinate dimer, N-isopropyl-p-123Iiodoamphetamine (IMP), and 123I-N,N,N'-trimethyl-N'-(2-hydroxy-3-methyl-5-iodobenzyl)-1,3-propanediamine (HIPDM). All of the currently available tracers closely follow 133Xe-derived regional cerebral blood flow values over the physiologic range.[42–44] HMPAO has many advantages, including but not limited to a low risk of allergic reaction, higher extraction, and a better signal-to-noise ratio. 125I-IMP is widely used outside the United States with excellent results.

OVERVIEW OF SINGLE-PHOTON EMISSION COMPUTED TOMOGRAPHY STUDIES IN TRAUMATIC BRAIN INJURY

A systematic review published in 2014 by Raji and colleagues[46] showed level IIA evidence (at least 1 randomized, controlled trial) for the usefulness of brain SPECT scanning in TBI. The review identified 52 cross-sectional and 19 longitudinal studies in a total of 2634 individuals over 30 years of literature supporting this conclusion. The majority of these studies focused on mTBI. One investigation of SPECT scanning by Abdel-Dayem et al[47] involving 228 patients identified abnormally low perfusion in the frontal, temporal, and parietal lobes. A follow-up study by Abu-Judeh et al[48] in the same population found that abnormalities on SPECT scanning were often not seen or were underestimated in magnitude on CT scan in those receiving both SPECT and CT scans. This finding is important because CT scans, although useful for revealing hemorrhage and fractures, will not show functional deficits seen on SPECT scanning, for which there may be no structural correlates. Additionally, although CT scans for head trauma in the emergency department may be negative, this finding does not rule out future functional deficits, particularly in cases of mTBI. Similarly, SPECT scanning is more sensitive for traumatic neural injury than anatomic MR imaging. In a series of 13 patients

with moderate TBI, Shin and colleagues[49] found that MR imaging was negative in 50% of the cases, whereas the SPECT scans were positive for brain injury in 100% of cases. Abu-Judeh et al[48] examined 228 patients with mild to moderate TBI in a retrospective review. Both CT and MR imaging within 2 weeks of injury were negative, whereas SPECT scans revealed frontal lobe injury in 24% of cases and temporal lobe injury in 13% of cases. Likewise, Stamatakis and colleagues[50] examined 62 TBI patients with MR imaging and SPECT scans performed within 2 weeks of injury. Using statistical parametric analysis, they found that SPECT scanning detected more lesions and more lesion volume than anatomic MR imaging.

In contrast, SPECT scanning has demonstrated excellent negative and positive predictive values. In a prospective evaluation of 136 patients by Jacobs and colleagues,[51] all patients had CT and SPECT scans within 2 weeks of injury and baseline neuropsychological testing. The CT scans of all patients were negative. Those patients with a negative baseline SPECT scan underwent repeat neuropsychological testing at 12 months. Those patients with a positive baseline SPECT scan underwent repeat SPECT scans and neuropsychological testing at 6 and at 12 months. A negative baseline SPECT scan was highly predictive of normal neuropsychological testing in the future. As shown in **Table 2**, SPECT scanning had a negative predictive value of 100% at 6 and 12 months after injury.[51] The main implication of this work is that a negative SPECT scan shortly after the initial injury predicts no long-term

Table 2
Sensitivity, specificity, positive predictive value, and negative predictive value of baseline SPECT

Months After TBI	0 (%)	3 (%)	6 (%)	12 (%)
Sensitivity	78	91	100	100
Specificity	61	61	53	85
Negative predictive value	92[a] 100[b]	89	100	100
Positive predictive value	44	64	52	83

Performed on a single-headed camera relative to neuropsychological testing, which was repeated at 3, 6, and 12 months after the injury. The negative predictive value at baseline is reported relative to performance on neuropsychological testing at [a]3 and [b]12 months.

Adapted from Jacobs A, Put E, Ingels M, et al. One-year follow-up of technetium-99m-HMPAO SPECT in mild head injury. J Nucl Med 1996;37(10):1605–9; with permission.

functional deficits. This finding cannot be said of other imaging modalities, such as conventional CT or MR imaging. In terms of positive predictive values, an abnormal baseline SPECT scanning had a sensitivity of 100% and specificity of 85% for predicting persistent neuropsychological deficits at 12 months.[51] Similarly, Laatsch and colleagues[52] found that an abnormal baseline SPECT scanning correlated strongly with abnormal neuropsychological testing in patients participating in a cognitive rehabilitation program. In total, 18 cross-sectional studies showed a correlation between abnormal SPECT findings and neuropsychological deficits.[46] This finding

suggests that abnormalities found with brain SPECT scanning can correlate with and, therefore, be predictive of functional outcomes.

In both cross-sectional and longitudinal SPECT studies of TBI, the frontal lobes are the most commonly identified abnormal regions.[47,48,50,52–74] Fig. 2 summarizes findings of the systematic review concerning lesion localization,[46] showing percentages of abnormal regions in SPECT studies on TBI superimposed on a volume-rendered normal SPECT image. After a TBI, the temporal lobes are the mostly frequently abnormal region on SPECT followed by the parietal and temporal lobes.

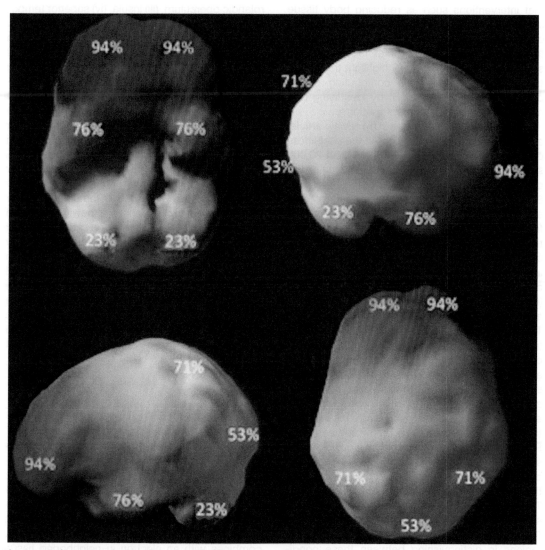

Fig. 2. A 3-dimensional rendered single-photon emission computed tomography (SPECT) scan with numbers representing percentage of low perfusion in the studies reviewed in reference.[46] For example, 94% of studies showed abnormal SPECT scans in traumatic brain injury in the frontal lobes. These same studies showed perfusion abnormalities in 76%, 71%, 53%, and 23% studies with SPECT data on the temporal, parietal, occipital, and cerebellar regions, respectively.

SPECT scanning also has been used to assess treatment outcomes in TBI. In the late nineties, Laatsch and colleagues[52,75] showed increased cerebral blood flow on serial SPECT scans in persons with TBI positively responding to cognitive behavioral therapy. Two studies used serial SPECT scans and showed that increases in perfusion paralleled response to hyperbaric oxygen therapy. The first study by Harch and colleagues[76] examined 13 patients who were exposed to blast injury 1 to 5 years before treatment, and the second study by Boussi-Gross et al[77] examined 56 patients at 1 to 5 years after mild TBI. Finally, a multifactorial lifestyle program in a cohort of retired NFL players by Amen and colleagues[78] showed that interventions such as reducing body tissue adiposity as reflected by reducing body mass index produced increases in SPECT cerebral blood flow, particularly in the frontal lobes.[69] These studies are significant as they highlight the importance of SPECT scans as contributing to the personalized medicine of TBI by identifying biomarkers that predict treatment response.

Since the publication of the 2014 review article, additional studies have highlighted the usefulness of SPECT in TBI. One study of more than 20,000 subjects showed that SPECT scanning can distinguish TBI from posttraumatic stress disorder with 80% to 100% sensitivity and an average of 70% specificity.[79] The study examined 2 groups. The first consisted of small samples (n = 104) of patients with TBI or posttraumatic stress disorder or those who had both (n = 73) closely matched in demographics and comorbidity with a well-characterized group of healthy controls (n = 116). The second group consisted of large and more diverse populations of patients with TBI (n = 7505), posttraumatic stress disorder (n = 1077), or both diagnoses (n = 1017) compared with a sample of patients with other diagnoses (n = 11,147). The second group represented a more real-world situation.[79] Both groups were subjected to visual reads by experienced clinicians and analyzed using a binary logistic regression model based on 14 cortical ROIs. Predicted probabilities from binary logistic regression models were then inputted into a receiver operating characteristic analysis. Replication of this study in a smaller study of 196 veterans with TBI, posttraumatic stress disorder, or both diagnoses showed an accuracy of between 83% and 94% of SPECT imaging of default mode network regions in distinguishing between these conditions.[80] This is particularly enlightening because the high accuracy, even in the comorbid cases, allows the separation of these 2 populations that overlap both in clinical history and symptoms.

Because TBI and posttraumatic stress disorder have very different treatment approaches, the accurate differentiation of these 2 populations is critical.[80] Consequently, SPECT scanning can contribute to personalized medicine approaches to better stratify treatment for posttraumatic stress disorder versus TBI.

SPECT scanning also continues to be used in sports-related TBI. One study published in the largest group of retired NFL players (n = 161) showed that SPECT regions alone allow for a diagnostic separation from controls with 94% accuracy, 90% sensitivity, and 86% specificity.[81] The most predictive regions underlying this separation were the (i) anterior superior temporal lobes, (ii) rolandic operculum, (iii) insula, (iv) superior temporal poles, (v) precuneus, and (vi) cerebellar vermis. The insula is of particular interest, because it is an important functional region in depression[82] and depression itself is a frequent symptom in football players who have sustained TBI.[83] The abnormality of the precuneus in this study is important because it is also abnormal in Alzheimer's disease[84] and TBI itself is an independent risk factor for Alzheimer's disease.[85] As imaging science in football and sports-related TBI evolves, SPECT scanning will be an important tool both for research and clinical applications.

Recent studies also confirm the usefulness for SPECT in tracking responses to newly developed treatments for TBI. Henderson and Morries[86] have shown that perfusion changes seen by SPECT correlated with clinical response to an innovative treatment for TBI with transcranial near infrared laser phototherapy, supporting clinical improvements seen in a case series.[87] Future studies with randomized, controlled clinical trials will be important for determining the highest level of evidence to support SPECT in such treatment applications (Fig. 3).

THE PHYSICS OF PET

PET imaging is based on the use of positron emitters linked to a radiopharmaceutical agent. PET uses gamma rays from positron emitters. Examples of such emitters are [11]carbon (half-life of 20 minutes) and fluorodeoxyglucose (^{18}F; half-life of 110 minutes). PET studies are typically done at rest and involve injection of positron emitters that then undergo an annihilation event in which a positron released by F-18, for example, combines with an electron in neighboring tissue and releases 2 gamma rays in opposite directions. PET scanners use coincidence detection to identify pairs of gamma rays to determine the location of annihilation events. PET scintillator crystals, the

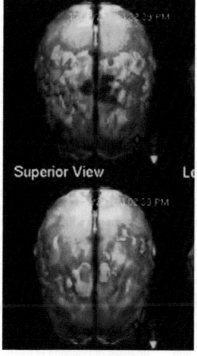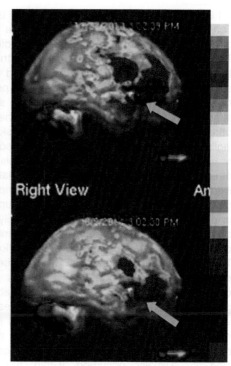

Before Treatment

After Treatment

Superior View   Right Lateral View

Fig. 3. Functional improvement after transcranial multi-Watt near-infrared phototherapy using quantitative analysis of single-photon emission computed tomography (SPECT) perfusion neuroimaging. A patient with moderate traumatic brain injury documented in anatomic MR imaging and perfusion SPECT received 20 near infrared treatments over the course of 2 months.[86] The area of anatomic injury is at the *blue arrow*. Areas of 4 to 6 standard deviations below the mean perfusion (cerebral blood flow) are shown in shades of *blue* and *black*. Areas of 2 to 3 standard deviations below the mean perfusion are shown in shades of *green*. Significant improvement in perfusion is demonstrated after this innovative treatment.

most common being Lu2SiO5:Ce, are used to convert gamma photons into visible light photons for subsequent detection by photomultiplier tubes. PET imaging thus depends on the visualization of the annihilation of a positron that has been released by the radiopharmaceutical. Current PET cameras depend on detection and triangulation of the energy burst that occurs at the time of the positron annihilation. This detection can be quite precise and much is made of the superior resolution of PET incidence detectors. Yet, there is a logical flaw. The detectors resolve the location of the annihilation of the positron, not the location where it was released from the radiopharmaceutical. A positron released from a radiopharmaceutical moves around in this process, losing energy colliding into electrons and molecules, causing secondary events before its annihilation. It has been estimated that an 800-kiloelectron volts (keV) positron produces an average of 32,000 ion pairs, leading to a considerable number of secondary events before its annihilation.[88] Eventually,

a positron loses enough energy to collide into an electron of identical energy and an annihilation event occurs. The mass of these 2 particles is converted into energy and a resulting 2 photons are giving off with exactly 511 keV of energy. Consequently, the movement range of positrons is up to 1 cm and the mean is about 3 mm, so the resolution is in the range of 4.5 mm[88]

OVERVIEW OF PET STUDIES IN TRAUMATIC BRAIN INJURY
Fluorodeoxyglucose

Fluorodeoxyglucose (FDG) is a PET radiopharmaceutical used to visualize and quantify metabolism. Imaging in FDG-PET scanning is the integration of FDG accumulation over 20 minutes. Thus, concentration tasks are often contaminated by periods of rest, because it is difficult to expect a person with a TBI or even a healthy individual to concentrate continuously over a 20-minute time period.

FDG-PET neuroimaging studies of mTBI or concussion have been limited with only a total of 60 subjects across all published studies.[89] The data are further fragmented because the interval since injury in these studies ranged from acute (days) to chronic (years). In addition, protocols were inconsistent. For example, some studies used "resting" or baseline scans whereas others used continuous performance tasks or vigilance tasks. Data analysis was also a source of variability with some using SUV analysis and others using relative uptake value (RUV) analysis. Because the ROI and RUV analysis compares glucose uptake in brain regions with the uptake in a designated reference region—typically the cerebellum—it is vulnerable to overestimation of regional glucose uptake in the situation of TBI if injury has occurred to the cerebellum directly or cross-cerebellar diaschisis has occurred. In each of these situations, cerebellar glucose uptake would be abnormally decreased, which artificially increases RUV values in other regions. One group has characterized an acute period of hyperglycolysis in the areas of contusion.[90,91] Usually occurring within the first 5 days after an injury, the disparity between perfusion and the metabolic rate may account for secondary pathophysiology, such as cortical spreading depression, changes in interstitial potassium and calcium, and subsequent spreading injury cascade.[1]

Early studies were generally retrospective case series with ROI. The first study described 3 patients with mTBI and decreased metabolism in the frontal and temporal lobes.[92] An early study of mTBI by Gross and colleagues[93] summarized 20 patients with mTBI and persistent neuropsychological symptoms. Decreased metabolism in the middle and anterior temporal, anterior cingulate, and precuneus cortices were most strongly associated with neuropsychological test results. Nakayama and colleagues[94] described 52 patients with severe TBI (n = 30 with impaired consciousness) using statistical parametric mapping and showed hypometabolism severity correlated with symptom severity. A second group found a similar correlation.[95] An interesting early finding that has significance for subsequent ROI analyses is that the cerebellar vermis is hypermetabolic in TBI. The case series of 58 patients with toxic brain injury, anoxic brain injury, or TBI showed elevated metabolism in the vermis with a ratio to the whole cerebellum of 1.27.[96] These early studies have been summarized by Dubroff and Newberg[97] and Lin and colleagues.[98]

Three FDG-PET studies of mTBI did not provide any quantification. Umile and colleagues[99]

examined 13 patients with mTBI using both SPECT perfusion neuroimaging and FDG-PET neuroimaging. Approximately 85% of the patients with mTBI had decreased perfusion and decreased metabolism in the frontal and temporal lobes. A single case study of an adult 2 days after a mTBI revealed no metabolic changes.[100] In contrast, a case study of an 11-year-old boy at approximately 2 years after injury revealed decreased metabolism in the temporal lobes and the cerebellum.[101] Zhang and colleagues[102] compared 81 patients with mTBI, including 41 with no findings on MR imaging or CT scans, with 68 controls using statistical parametric analysis. The frontal and temporal lobes bilaterally were most commonly affected, but multiple areas were involved reflecting the diversity of injury. There is a paucity of studies comparing FDG-PET findings to neuropsychological testing results.

Studies of blast-related concussion or mTBI have suggested a somewhat different pattern of injury. Peskind and colleagues[103] described 12 veterans with repetitive blast exposures. An RUV analysis of baseline FDG-PET revealed decreased metabolism in the cerebellum, pons, and medial temporal cortex as the strongest correlates of persistent symptoms.[103] A larger study of baseline FDG-PET in 12 veterans with repetitive blast exposure used an RUV analysis as well.[104] A unique finding among blast-exposed subjects was a decreased right superior parietal cortex metabolism. Involvement of the inferior frontal, inferolateral temporal, posterior cingulate, and left thalamus also was described. The strongest correlate of persistent neurocognitive symptoms was decreased metabolism in the left medial frontal cortex. Petrie and colleagues[105] compared 34 veterans with blast exposure with 18 veterans without history of blast exposure. Decreased metabolism was found in the parietal, right visual, and left sensory cortex, and in the parahippocampal gyri. In a review article, Byrnes and colleagues[89] described decreased frontal lobe metabolisms in single cases of blast-exposed veterans. This work has been summarized by Wintermark and colleagues[106] and Hetherington and colleagues.[107] An early study of 19 boxers who suffered repetitive concussive blows to the head[108] showed a pattern of decreased metabolism in the superior parietal and parietooccipital cortices, as well as the posterior cingulate cortex, frontal lobes, and cerebellum. The involvement of parietal and posterior cingulate cortices is quite similar to findings in recent studies of blast injury. This involvement raises a question as to the specificity of these findings or blast-induced TBI.

Emerging molecular PET tracers

Although molecular PET with amyloid and tau imaging has been applied in a limited number of professional football players with suspected CTE,[109] this approach is not approved by the US Food and Drug Administration at this time. However, this area continues to be a focus of active research. Because CTE is believed to be a secondary tauopathy, according to Villemagne and colleagues'[110] application of tau PET imaging holds potential as a tool for adding specificity to the diagnosis. The importance of such a biomarker is critical as tau is better linked to cognitive decline than other molecular biomarkers for neurodegeneration, such as amyloid.[111] Sundman and colleagues[112] review a variety of modalities in mTBI in which tau imaging is again highlighted as a possible confirmatory test for abnormalities detected in multiparametric MR imaging sequences.

INTEGRATION OF SINGLE-PHOTON EMISSION COMPUTED TOMOGRAPHY INTO THE ASSESSMENT OF TRAUMATIC BRAIN INJURY

The most current recommendations of the American College of Radiology for assessment of head trauma in adults and children focus on use of structural neuroimaging modalities (CT and MR imaging).[113,114] To quote these recommendations with respect to advanced neuroimaging modalities such as SPECT:

Advanced neuroimaging techniques (SPECT, PET, perfusion CT and MRI, DTI, functional MRI, and MRS) are areas of active research but are not considered routine clinical practice at this time.[113]

Given that functional changes are more sensitive to changes in TBI compared with structural changes,[115] a functional imaging method will eventually be applied in the routine clinical assessment of TBI. SPECT imaging is well-positioned to be one such option owing to its availability in and outpatient setting and more importantly owing to the large amount of imaging data that already exist.[53] A recent report described at least 14,825 SPECT scanners performing an estimated 14.5 million imaging procedures per year from 2008 to 2012.[116] For PET, there are about 1600 scanners performing about 1.5 million scans per year.[117] Thus, from a patient access standpoint there is greater ability for SPECT to be leveraged for functional neuroimaging evaluations in TBI. The large number of images acquirable from such availability of SPECT scanners can also be used to power application of

artificial intelligence algorithms that can provided personalized prediction of outcomes in TBI.[118] Such large databases are still being developed for other advanced imaging modalities. Other limitations also exist. PET scans, as discussed, are of high expense ranging from $1266.40 with FDG PET to $2721.83 for molecular imaging with amyloid PET.[119] Brain SPECT imaging is the least expensive neuronuclear modality with a total cost of $1025.86 for the CPT code of 78607, based on Health and Human Services reimbursement. According to New Choice Health, which provides transparency in health costs for many procedures, an FDG-PET can cost from $2000 to $6000, depending on location.[120] Perfusion CT scanning has radiation exposure comparable with SPECT scanning[121] and thus presents no major advantage from a radiation standpoint. Perfusion MR imaging is quite appealing owing to the lack of exposure to ionizing radiation, but no known head-to-head comparisons with SPECT have been done in TBI. One study done in Alzheimer's disease showed SPECT scanning had a superior area under the curve, on average of 10% higher in identifying Alzheimer's disease compared with ASL MR imaging.[122] Whether or not such a result would be observed in a TBI comparison study would be an important subject of future investigation. Functional MR imaging, as discussed, has encountered issues with postprocessing rendering that can limit insight gleaned from such studies,[45] but remains potentially promising for future development. MR spectroscopy has shown low metabolite concentration of *N*-acetylaspartate in mTBI, but the anatomic specificity of these findings is unclear given the limited studies done in this area.[123] Diffusion tensor imaging will be important for better characterization of structural imaging findings and generating connectome models[124] that would benefit from inclusion of perfusion data from SPECT. Ultimately, multimodal approaches will be important, integrating perfusion SPECT scans with other modalities for the maximal benefit to patient care.[125]

SUMMARY

SPECT and PET scans are 2 neuronuclear imaging techniques that have been applied to TBI, particularly mTBI. Of the 2 methods, more literature has been published on SPECT. Both methods will continue to be important as the science of neuroimaging in TBI continues to advance. Of note, the radiopharmaceuticals for SPECT perfusion imaging are widely available and approved by federal pharmaceutical regulatory agencies.

In contrast, radiopharmaceuticals for PET, which depend on a cyclotron for production and are generally short lived, are considerably less available and not approved by the US Food and Drug Administration or equivalent bodies in other countries. Moreover, the cost of an FDG-PET scan is generally twice that of a perfusion SPECT scan. Coupled with the limited availability of PET imaging centers compared with the relative abundance of SPECT cameras, a SPECT scan is a more affordable and readily available neuronuclear procedure for examining TBI. Given the shortcomings of postprocessing metrics in functional MR imaging and the recent advances in SPECT quantitative analysis, SPECT offers a promising opportunity to assess TBI, even mTBI, and provide both screening and postinjury monitoring quantitative data.

REFERENCES

1. Bigler ED, Maxwell WL. Neuropathology of mild traumatic brain injury: relationship to neuroimaging findings. Brain Imaging Behav 2012;6(2):108–36.
2. Peskind ER, Brody D, Cernak I, et al. Military- and sports-related mild traumatic brain injury: clinical presentation, management, and long-term consequences. J Clin Psychiatry 2013;74(2):180–8.
3. Humphreys I, Wood RL, Phillips CJ, et al. The costs of traumatic brain injury: a literature review. Clinicoecon Outcomes Res 2013;5:281.
4. Gessel LM, Fields SK, Collins CL, et al. Concussions among United States high school and collegiate athletes. J Athl Train 2007;42(4):495–503.
5. Covassin T, Moran R, Wilhelm K. Concussion symptoms and neurocognitive performance of high school and college athletes who incur multiple concussions. Am J Sports Med 2013;41(12):2885–9.
6. Peschman J, Neideen T, Brasel K. The impact of discharging minimally injured trauma patient. J Trauma 2011;70(6):1331–5.
7. Richmond R, Aldaghlas TA, Burke C, et al. Age: is it all in the head? Factors influencing mortality in elderly patients with head injuries. J Trauma 2011;71(1):E8–11.
8. Ramanathan DM, McWilliams N, Schatz P, et al. Epidemiological shifts in elderly traumatic brain injury: 18-year trends in Pennsylvania. J Neurotrauma 2012;29(7):1371–8.
9. Susman M, DiRusso SM, Sullivan T, et al. Traumatic brain injury in the elderly: increased mortality and worse functional outcome at discharge despite lower injury severity. J Trauma 2002;53(2):219–23.
10. Wong GK, Tang BYH, Yeung JHH, et al. Traumatic intracerebral haemorrhage: is the CT pattern related to outcome? Br J Neurosurg 2009;23(6):601–5.
11. Styrke J, Stålnacke BM, Sojka P, et al. Traumatic brain injuries in a well-defined population: epidemiological aspects and severity. J Neurotrauma 2007;24(9):1425–36.
12. Shapey J, Glancz LJ, Brennan PM. Chronic subdural haematoma in the elderly: is it time for a new paradigm in management? Curr Geriatr Rep 2016;5:71–7.
13. Cobb BR, Urban JE, Davenport EM, et al. Head impact exposure in youth football: elementary school ages 9–12 years and the effect of practice structure. Ann Biomed Eng 2013;41(12):2463–73.
14. Urban JE, Davenport EM, Golman AJ, et al. Head impact exposure in youth football: high school ages 14 to 18 years and cumulative impact analysis. Ann Biomed Eng 2013;41(12):2474–87.
15. Omalu BI, DeKosky ST, Minster RL, et al. Chronic traumatic encephalopathy in a national football league player. Neurosurgery 2005;57(1):128–34.
16. Omalu B, Bailes J, Hamilton RL, et al. Emerging histomorphologic phenotypes of chronic traumatic encephalopathy in American athletes. Neurosurgery 2011;69(1):173–83.
17. McKee AC, Cantu RC, Nowinski CJ, et al. Chronic traumatic encephalopathy in athletes: progressive tauopathy after repetitive head injury. J Neuropathol Exp Neurol 2009;68(7):709–35.
18. Pennington B. C.T.E. Is found in an ex-Giant Tyler Sash, who died at 27. The New York Times 2016.
19. Grubenhoff JA, Deakyne SJ, Brou L, et al. Acute concussion symptom severity and delayed symptom resolution. Pediatrics 2014;134(1):54–62.
20. Stamm JM, Bourlas AP, Baugh CM, et al. Age of first exposure to football and later-life cognitive impairment in former NFL players. Neurology 2015;84(11):1114.
21. RADAR Home. Available at: http://www.doseinfo-radar.com/. Accessed January 31, 2017.
22. United States Environmental Protection Agency (EPA). Radiation protection: calculate your radiation dose website. Available at: https://www.epa.gov/radiation/calculate-your-radiation-dose. Accessed January 31, 2017.
23. Howe GR, McLaughlin J. Breast cancer mortality between 1950 and 1987 after exposure to fractionated moderate-dose-rate ionizing radiation in the Canadian fluoroscopy cohort study and a comparison with breast cancer mortality in the atomic bomb survivors study. Radiat Res 1996;145(6):694–707.
24. National Research Council (US) Committee on Health Effects of Exposure to Low Levels of Ionizing Radiations (BEIR VII). Health effects of exposure to low levels of ionizing radiations: time

for reassessment? Washington, DC: National Academies Press (US); 1998.

25. Cohen BL. The cancer risk from low level radiation: a review of recent evidence. Med Sentinel 2000; 5(4):128–31.

26. Cardis E, Gilbert ES, Carpenter L, et al. Effects of low doses and low dose rates of external ionizing radiation: cancer mortality among nuclear industry workers in three countries. Radiat Res 1995;142(2): 117–32.

27. Health Physics Society (HPS). Radiation risk in perspective: position statement of the health physics society. Available at: https://hps.org/documents/risk_ps010-2.pdf. Accessed January 31, 2017.

28. American Nuclear Society Position Statement #41. Health effects of low-level radiation. ANS/Public Information. Available at: http://cdn.ans.org/pi/ps/docs/ps41.pdf. Accessed January 31, 2017.

29. American Cancer Society. Cancer facts & figures 2010. Available at: https://www.cancer.org/research/cancer-facts-statistics/all-cancer-facts-figures/cancer-facts-figures-2010.html. Accessed January 31, 2017.

30. Saenger EL, Thoma GE, Tompkins EA. Incidence of leukemia following treatment of hyperthyroidism: preliminary report of the cooperative thyrotoxicosis therapy follow-up study. JAMA 1968;205(12): 855–62.

31. Ron E, Modan B. Benign and malignant thyroid neoplasms after childhood irradiation for tinea capitis. J Natl Cancer Inst 1980;65(1):7–11.

32. Ernst M, Freed ME, Zametkin AJ. Health hazards of radiation exposure in the context of brain imaging research: special consideration for children. J Nucl Med 1998;39(4):689–98.

33. Devous MD. SPECT functional brain imaging. In: Toga AW, Mazziotta JC, editors. Brain map. Methods. 2nd edition. London: Academic Press; 2002. p. 513–36.

34. Devous MD. SPECT functional brain imaging: instrumentation, radiopharmaceuticals, and technical factors. In: Van Heertum RL, Tikovsky RS, Ichise M, editors. Functional cerebral SPECT and PET imaging. 4th edition. Philadelphia: Wolter Kluwer Lippincott Williams & Wilkins; 2010. p. 3–22.

35. Harkness LJ, Boston AJ, Boston HC, et al. Prospectus: development of a Compton camera for medical imaging. In: Dössel O, Schlegel WC, editors. World Congress on medical physics and Biomedical Engineering, September 7-12, 2009, Munich, Germany. Cham (Switzerland): Springer International Publishing AG; 2009. p. 102–5.

36. Liu CJ, Cheng JS, Chen YC, et al. A performance comparison of novel cadmium-zinc-telluride camera and conventional SPECT/CT using

anthropomorphic torso phantom and water bags to simulate soft tissue and breast attenuation. Ann Nucl Med 2015;29(4):342–50.

37. Takahashi Y, Miyagawa M, Nishiyama Y, et al. Performance of a semiconductor SPECT system: comparison with a conventional Anger-type SPECT instrument. Ann Nucl Med 2013;27(1): 11–6.

38. Kinahan PE, Fletcher JW. PET/CT standardized uptake values (SUVs) in clinical practice and assessing response to therapy. Semin Ultrasound CT MR 2010;31(6):496–505.

39. Foster B, Bagci U, Mansoor A, et al. A review on segmentation of positron emission tomography images. Comput Biol Med 2014;0:76–96.

40. Hill TC, Costello P, Gramm HF, et al. Early clinical experience with a radionuclide emission computed tomographic brain imaging system. Radiology 1978;128(3):803–6.

41. Shin SS, Bales JW, Edward Dixon C, et al. Structural imaging of mild traumatic brain injury may not be enough: overview of functional and metabolic imaging of mild traumatic brain injury. Brain Imaging Behav 2017;11(2):591–610.

42. Devous Michael D. SPECT functional brain imaging; technical considerations. J Neuroimaging 1995;5(Suppl 1):S2–13.

43. Darcourt J, Mena I, Cauvin J-C, et al. Absolute calibration of HMPAO SPECT using (133)Xe rCBF values. Alasbimn J 1999;2(5).

44. Payne JK, Trivedi MH, Devous MD Sr. Comparison of technetium-99m-HMPAO and xenon-133 measurements of regional cerebral blood flow by SPECT. J Nucl Med 1996;37(10):1735–40.

45. Eklund A, Nichols TE, Knutsson H. Cluster failure: why fMRI inferences for spatial extent have inflated false-positive rates. Proc Natl Acad Sci U S A 2016; 113(28):7900–5.

46. Raji CA, Tarzwell R, Pavel D, et al. Clinical utility of SPECT neuroimaging in the diagnosis and treatment of traumatic brain injury: a systematic review. PLoS One 2014;9(3):e91088.

47. Abdel-Dayem HM, Abu-Judeh H, Kumar M, et al. SPECT brain perfusion abnormalities in mild or moderate traumatic brain injury. Clin Nucl Med 1998;23(5):309–17.

48. Abu-Judeh HH, Parker R, Aleksic S, et al. SPECT brain perfusion findings in mild or moderate traumatic brain injury. Nucl Med Rev Cent East Eur 2000;3(1):5–11.

49. Shin YB, Kim S-J, Kim I-J, et al. Voxel-based statistical analysis of cerebral blood flow using Tc-99m ECD brain SPECT in patients with traumatic brain injury: group and individual analyses. Brain Inj 2006;20(6):661–7.

50. Stamatakis EA, Wilson JT, Hadley DM, et al. SPECT imaging in head injury interpreted with statistical

parametric mapping. J Nucl Med 2002;43(4): 476–83.

51. Jacobs A, Put E, Ingels M, et al. One-year follow-up of technetium-99m-HMPAO SPECT in mild head injury. J Nucl Med 1996;37(10):1605–9.

52. Laatsch L, Jobe T, Sychra J, et al. Impact of cognitive rehabilitation therapy on neuropsychological impairments as measured by brain perfusion SPECT: a longitudinal study. Brain Inj 1997; 11(12):851–63.

53. Amen DG, Willeumier K. Brain SPECT imaging: a powerful, evidence-based tool for transforming clinical psychiatric practice. Minerva Psichiatr 2011;52:109–23.

54. Assadi M, Eftekhari M, Gholamrezanezhad A. SPET brain scan with (99m)Tc-ECD and CT, MRI in traumatic brain injury with chronic symptoms. Hell J Nucl Med 2007;10(3):183.

55. Audenaert K, Jansen HM, Otte A, et al. Imaging of mild traumatic brain injury using 57Co and 99mTc HMPAO SPECT as compared to other diagnostic procedures. Med Sci Monit 2003;9(10):MT112–7.

56. Bicik I, Radanov BP, Schafer N, et al. PET with 18fluorodeoxyglucose and hexamethylpropylene amine oxime SPECT in late whiplash syndrome. Neurology 1998;51(2):345–50.

57. Bonne O, Gilboa A, Louzoun Y, et al. Cerebral blood flow in chronic symptomatic mild traumatic brain injury. Psychiatry Res 2003;124(3):141–52.

58. Cusumano S, Paolin A, Di Paola F, et al. Assessing brain function in post-traumatic coma by means of bit-mapped SEPs, BAEPs, CT, SPET and clinical scores. Prognostic implications. Electroencephalogr Clin Neurophysiol 1992;84(6):499–514.

59. Donnemiller E, Brenneis C, Wissel J, et al. Impaired dopaminergic neurotransmission in patients with traumatic brain injury: a SPECT study using 123I-beta-CIT and 123I-IBZM. Eur J Nucl Med 2000; 27(9):1410–4.

60. Goethals I, Audenaert K, Jacobs F, et al. Cognitive neuroactivation using SPECT and the Stroop colored word test in patients with diffuse brain injury. J Neurotrauma 2004;21(8):1059–69.

61. Goldenberg G, Oder W, Spatt J, et al. Cerebral correlates of disturbed executive function and memory in survivors of severe closed head injury: a SPECT study. J Neurol Neurosurg Psychiatry 1992;55(5): 362–8.

62. Goshen E, Zwas ST, Shahar E, et al. The role of 99Tcm-HMPAO brain SPECT in paediatric traumatic brain injury. Nucl Med Commun 1996;17(5): 418–22.

63. Gray BG, Ichise M, Chung DG, et al. Technetium-99m-HMPAO SPECT in the evaluation of patients with a remote history of traumatic brain injury: a comparison with x-ray computed tomography. J Nucl Med 1992;33(1):52–8.

64. Hashimoto K, Abo M. Abnormal regional benzodiazepine receptor uptake in the prefrontal cortex in patients with mild traumatic brain injury. J Rehabil Med 2009;41(8):661–5.

65. Hattori N, Swan M, Stobbe GA, et al. Differential SPECT activation patterns associated with PASAT performance may indicate frontocerebellar functional dissociation in chronic mild traumatic brain injury. J Nucl Med 2009;50(7):1054–61.

66. Hofman PA, Stapert SZ, van Kroonenburgh MJ, et al. MR imaging, single-photon emission CT, and neurocognitive performance after mild traumatic brain injury. AJNR Am J Neuroradiol 2001; 22(3):441–9.

67. Ichise M, Chung DG, Wang P, et al. Technetium-99m-HMPAO SPECT, CT and MRI in the evaluation of patients with chronic traumatic brain injury: a correlation with neuropsychological performance. J Nucl Med 1994;35(2):217–26.

68. Ito H, Kanno I, Ibaraki M, et al. Effect of aging on cerebral vascular response to Paco2 changes in humans as measured by positron emission tomography. J Cereb Blood Flow Metab 2002;22(8): 997–1003.

69. Jian X, Junyu W, Jinfang L. Post-traumatic mutism in children. Brain Inj 2009;23(5):445–9.

70. Kant R, Smith-Seemiller L, Isaac G, et al. Tc-HMPAO SPECT in persistent post-concussion syndrome after mild head injury: comparison with MRI/CT. Brain Inj 1997;11(2):115–24.

71. Kinuya K, Kakuda K, Nobata K, et al. Role of brain perfusion single-photon emission tomography in traumatic head injury. Nucl Med Commun 2004; 25(4):333–7.

72. Korn A, Golan H, Melamed I, et al. Focal cortical dysfunction and blood-brain barrier disruption in patients with Postconcussion syndrome. J Clin Neurophysiol 2005;22(1):1–9.

73. Sakas DE, Bullock MR, Patterson J, et al. Focal cerebral hyperemia after focal head injury in humans: a benign phenomenon? J Neurosurg 1995;83(2): 277–84.

74. Sataloff RT, Mandel S, Muscal E, et al. Single-photon-emission computed tomography (SPECT) in neurotologic assessment: a preliminary report. Am J Otol 1996;17(6):909–16.

75. Laatsch L, Pavel D, Jobe T, et al. Incorporation of SPECT imaging in a longitudinal cognitive rehabilitation therapy programme. Brain Inj 1999;13(8): 555–70.

76. Harch PG, Andrews SR, Fogarty EF, et al. A phase I study of low-pressure hyperbaric oxygen therapy for blast-induced post-concussion syndrome and post-traumatic stress disorder. J Neurotrauma 2012;29(1):168–85.

77. Boussi-Gross R, Golan H, Fishlev G, et al. Hyperbaric oxygen therapy can improve post

concussion syndrome years after mild traumatic brain injury - randomized prospective trial. PLoS One 2013;8(11):e79995.

78. Amen DG, Wu JC, Taylor D, et al. Reversing brain damage in former NFL players: implications for traumatic brain injury and substance abuse rehabilitation. J Psychoactive Drugs 2011;43(1):1–5.

79. Amen DG, Raji CA, Willeumier K, et al. Functional neuroimaging distinguishes posttraumatic stress disorder from traumatic brain injury in focused and large community datasets. PLoS One 2015; 10(7):e0129659.

80. Raji CA, Willeumier K, Taylor D, et al. Functional neuroimaging with default mode network regions distinguishes PTSD from TBI in a military veteran population. Brain Imaging Behav 2015;9(3): 527–34.

81. Amen DG, Willeumier K, Omalu B, et al. Perfusion neuroimaging abnormalities alone distinguish national football league players from a healthy population. J Alzheimers Dis 2016;53(1):237–41.

82. McGrath CL, Kelley ME, Holtzheimer PE, et al. Toward a neuroimaging treatment selection biomarker for major depressive disorder. JAMA Psychiatry 2013;70(8):821–9.

83. Pryor J, Larson A, DeBeliso M. The prevalence of depression and concussions in a sample of active North American semi-professional and professional football players. J Lifestyle Med 2016; 6(1):7.

84. Cavanna AE, Trimble M. The precuneus: a review of its functional anatomy and behavioral correlates. Brain 2006;129:564–83.

85. Veitch DP, Friedl KE, Weiner MW. Military risk factors for cognitive decline, dementia and Alzheimer's Disease. Available at: http://www.eurekaselect.com/113942/article. Accessed January 31, 2017, n.d.

86. Henderson TA, Morries LD. SPECT perfusion imaging demonstrates improvement of traumatic brain injury with transcranial near-infrared laser phototherapy. Adv Mind Body Med 2015;29(4):27–33.

87. Morries LD, Cassano P, Henderson TA. Treatments for traumatic brain injury with emphasis on transcranial near-infrared laser phototherapy. Neuropsychiatr Dis Treat 2015;11:2159–75.

88. Cherry SR, Phelps ME. Positron emission tomography: methods and instrumentation. In: Dandler MP, Coleman RE, Patton JA, et al, editors. Diagnostic nuclear medicine. 4th edition. Philadelphia: Lippincott Williams & Wilkins; 2003.

89. Byrnes KR, Wilson CM, Brabazon F, et al. FDG-PET imaging in mild traumatic brain injury: a critical review. Front Neuroenergetics 2014;5:13.

90. Wu H-M, Huang S-C, Vespa P, et al. Redefining the pericontusional penumbra following traumatic brain injury: evidence of deteriorating metabolic derangements based on positron emission tomography. J Neurotrauma 2013;30(5):352.

91. Bergschneider M, Hovda DA, Shalmon E. Cerebral hyperglycolysis following severe human traumatic brain injury: a positron emission tomography study. J Neurosurg 2003;86:241–51.

92. Humayun MS, Presty SK, Lafrance ND, et al. Local cerebral glucose abnormalities in mild closed head injured patients with cognitive impairments. Nucl Med Commun 1989;10(5):335–44.

93. Gross H, Kling A, Henry G, et al. Local cerebral glucose metabolism in patients with long- term behavioral and cognitive deficits following mild traumatic brain injury. J Neuropsychiatry Clin Neurosci 1996;8:324–34.

94. Nakayama N, Okumura A, Shinoda J, et al. Relationship between regional cerebral metabolism and consciousness disturbance in traumatic diffuse brain injury without large focal lesions: an FDG-PET study with statistical parametric mapping analysis. J Neurol Neurosurg Psychiatry 2006; 77(7):856.

95. García-Panach J, Lull N, Lull JJ, et al. A voxel-based analysis of FDG-PET in traumatic brain injury: regional metabolism and relationship between the thalamus and cortical areas. J Neurotrauma 2011;28(9):1707–17.

96. Lupi A, Bertagnoni G, Salgarello M, et al. Cerebellar vermis relative hypermetabolism: an almost constant PET finding in an injured brain. Clin Nucl Med 2007;32(6):445–51.

97. Dubroff J, Newberg A. Neuroimaging of traumatic brain injury. Semin Neurol 2008;28(4):548–57.

98. Lin AP, Liao HJ, Merugumala SK, et al. Metabolic imaging of mild traumatic brain injury. Brain Imaging Behav 2012;6(2):208–23.

99. Umile EM, Plotkin RC, Sandel ME. Functional assessment of mild traumatic brain injury using SPECT and neuropsychological testing. Brain Inj 1998;12(7):577–94.

100. Abu-Judeh HH, Singh M, Masdeu JC, et al. Discordance between FDG uptake and technetium-99m-HMPAO brain perfusion in acute traumatic brain injury. J Nucl Med 1998;39(8):1357–9.

101. Roberts MA, Manshadi FF, Bushnell DL, et al. Neurobehavioural dysfunction following mild traumatic brain injury in childhood: a case report with positive findings on positron emission tomography (PET). Brain Inj 1995;9(5):427–36.

102. Zhang J, Mitsis EM, Chu K, et al. Statistical parametric mapping and cluster counting analysis of [18 F] FDG-PET imaging in traumatic brain injury. J Neurotrauma 2010;27(1):35–49.

103. Peskind ER, Petrie EC, Cross DJ, et al. Cerebrocerebellar hypometabolism associated with repetitive blast exposure mild traumatic brain injury in 12 Iraq war Veterans with persistent

post-concussive symptoms. Neuroimage 2011; 54(Suppl 1):S76–82.

104. Mendez MF, Owens EM, Reza Berenji G, et al. Mild traumatic brain injury from primary blast vs. blunt forces: post-concussion consequences and functional neuroimaging. NeuroRehabilitation 2013; 32(2):397–407.

105. Petrie EC, Cross DJ, Yarnykh VL, et al. Neuroimaging, behavioral, and psychological sequelae of repetitive combined blast/impact mild traumatic brain injury in Iraq and Afghanistan War Veterans. J Neurotrauma 2014;31(5):425.

106. Wintermark M, Coombs L, Druzgal TJ, et al. Traumatic brain injury imaging research roadmap. AJNR Am J Neuroradiol 2015;36(3):E12–23.

107. Hetherington H, Bandak A, Ling G, et al. Advances in imaging explosive blast mild traumatic brain injury. Handb Clin Neurol 2015;127:309–18. Elsevier.

108. Provenzano FA, Jordan B, Tikofsky RS, et al. F-18 FDG PET imaging of chronic traumatic brain injury in boxers: a statistical parametric analysis. Nucl Med Commun 2010;31(11):952–7.

109. Barrio JR, Small GW, Wong KP, et al. In vivo characterization of chronic traumatic encephalopathy using [F-18]FDDNP PET brain imaging. Proc Natl Acad Sci U S A 2015;112(16): E2039–47.

110. Villemagne VL, Okamura N. Tau imaging in the study of ageing, Alzheimer's disease, and other neurodegenerative conditions. Curr Opin Neurobiol 2016;36:43–51.

111. Menon PM, Vonsattel JP, Jolles PR. Brain imaging and neuropathologic mechanisms in Alzheimer's Disease: vascular versus neurodegenerative and Amyloid-β Versus Tau. J Alzheimers Dis 2009; 18(2):419–27.

112. Sundman MH, Hall EE, Chen NK. Examining the relationship between head trauma and neurodegenerative disease: a review of epidemiology, pathology and neuroimaging techniques. J Alzheimers Dis Parkinsonism 2014;4 [pii:137].

113. Shetty VS, Reis MN, Aulino JM, et al. ACR appropriateness criteria head trauma. J Am Coll Radiol 2016;13(6):668–79.

114. Ryan ME, Palasis S, Saigal G, et al. ACR appropriateness criteria head trauma—child. J Am Coll Radiol 2014,11(10):939–47.

115. Eierud C, Craddock RC, Fletcher S, et al. Neuroimaging after mild traumatic brain injury: review and meta-analysis. Neuroimage Clin 2014;4: 283–94.

116. IMV Medical Information Division. IMV 2013 Nuclear Medicine Market Outlook Report. 2013.

117. Delbeke D, Segall GM. Status of and trends in nuclear medicine in the United States. J Nucl Med 2011;52(Supplement_2):24S–8S.

118. Lee SW, O'Doherty JP, Shimojo S. Neural computations mediating one-shot learning in the human brain. PLoS Biol 2015;13(4):e1002137.

119. Desikan RS, Rafii MS, Brewer JB, et al. An expanded role for neuroimaging in the evaluation of memory impairment. AJNR Am J Neuroradiol 2013;34(11):2075–82.

120. New Health Choice website. Available at: https:// www.newchoicehealth.com/. Accessed August 22, 2017.

121. Ringelstein A, Lechel U, Fahrendorf DM, et al. Radiation exposure in perfusion CT of the brain. J Comput Assist Tomogr 2014;38(1):25–8.

122. Takahashi H, Ishii K, Hosokawa C, et al. Clinical application of 3D arterial spin-labeled brain perfusion imaging for Alzheimer Disease: comparison with brain perfusion SPECT. Am J Neuroradiol 2014;35(5):906–11.

123. Wu X, Kirov II, Gonen O, et al. MR imaging applications in mild traumatic brain injury: an imaging update. Radiology 2016;279(3):693–707.

124. Owen JP, Wang MB, Mukherjee P. Periventricular white matter is a nexus for network connectivity in the human brain. Brain Connect 2016;6(7):548–57.

125. Lewine JD, Davis JT, Bigler ED, et al. Objective documentation of traumatic brain injury subsequent to mild head trauma: multimodal brain imaging with MEG, SPECT, and MRI. J Head Trauma Rehabil 2007;22(3):141–55.

Imaging the Role of Myelin in Concussion

Alexander Mark Weber, MSc, PhD[a,*], Carlos Torres, MD, FRCPC[b,c], Alexander Rauscher, MSc, PhD[a]

KEYWORDS

• Myelin water imaging • Mild traumatic brain injury • White matter • Brain

KEY POINTS

• Myelin water imaging (MWI) provides mild traumatic brain injury (mTBI) researchers with a specific myelin biomarker and helps to further elucidate microstructural and microarchitectural changes of white matter after mTBI.

• Ongoing improvement of scanner hardware and software with the implementation of MWI across scanner platforms will likely result in increased research regarding the role of myelin in traumatic brain injury.

• Initial results show altered myelin 2 weeks after concussion and normalization by 2 months after injury.

INTRODUCTION

Myelin, the fatty substance that surrounds, protects, and electrically insulates axons in the central nervous system, is thought to play an important role in the pathophysiology of mild traumatic brain injuries (mTBIs).[1,2] White matter tracts (both myelinated and nonmyelinated axons) are vulnerable to damage from the impact-acceleration forces sustained in a traumatic brain injury (TBI), with evidence indicating that nonmyelinated axons are more vulnerable than myelinated ones.[3] Further evidence suggests that damage to either the axon or myelin sheath alone can lead to damage to the other.[4,5] This damage occurs from diffuse shear strains caused by linear and rotational acceleration of the brain during blast impacts. As opposed to more severe TBI, in which complete axon severance is observed following high-magnitude impacts, it is thought that axonal and myelin disorder in mTBI takes days to weeks

to develop.[6–10] After primary axonal shearing and stretching, and possible blood capillary ruptures,[6] a cascade of secondary mechanisms takes place through biochemical, metabolic, and cellular changes.[10] Briefly, these changes include an increased sodium influx, which results in a continuously working sodium-potassium pump to restore the resting state of the neurons. More energy in the form of adenosine triphosphate is required and this is measurable through an increased blood flow. During the acute stage of mTBI, around 48 hours, the brain first experiences this increased blood flow and is able to compensate for the high energy demand.[10] However, shortly afterward, over the subsequent 24 hours, the cerebral perfusion becomes diminished, leading to an insufficient energy supply.[10] This reduction in global and regional blood flow has been linked to recovery duration,[11] with some work suggesting a subsequent oxidative stress

Disclosures: The authors report no disclosure.
[a] Department of Pediatrics, Division of Neurology, Faculty of Medicine, University of British Columbia, M10 - Purdy Pavilion, 2221 Wesbrook Mall, Vancouver, British Columbia V6T 2B5, Canada; [b] Department of Radiology, University of Ottawa, 1053 Carling Avenue, Ottawa, Ontario K1Y 4E9, Canada; [c] Department of Medical Imaging, The Ottawa Hospital, 1053 Carling Avenue, Ottawa, Ontario K1Y 4E9, Canada
* Corresponding author.
E-mail address: alex.weber@ubc.ca

accumulation that results in suppression of the differentiation of oligodendrocyte precursor cells to oligodendrocytes, as well as myelin renewal.[12] This process in turn is expected to lead to a loss of oligodendrocytes and demyelination of the axons.[2,5,13] A second injury during this vulnerable period of reduced blood flow can result in even more serious injuries.[14] Along with the ionic flux, indiscriminate glutamate release occurs, leading to mitochondrial dysfunction and calcium sequestration, further exasperating the energy crisis and causing cytoskeletal damage.[10] Damage to the myelin and oligodendrocytes can occur through this calcium overload in the cytoplasm.[15] Swelling of the axon caused by impaired transport can lead to axonal disconnection and wallerian degeneration (anterograde degeneration).[6,16] These observations have been seen in histopathology specimens, showing axonal bulbs, irregular tortuous axonal swellings, and small sections of degraded myelin sheaths.[1,17,18]

Myelin Damage in Mild Traumatic Brain Injury

Myelin damage observations in mTBI have come in the form of decompaction, fragmentation, and complete degradation.[1,17,19–22] A study by Johnson and colleagues[19] provided evidence for myelin degeneration and active phagocytosis of myelin fragments in humans following moderate/severe TBI. Donovan and colleagues[23] showed that repeated mTBI in rats leads to a spectrum of changes, including separation of the myelin sheath from the axon, decompaction of the myelin sheath, and fragmentation of the myelin sheath. In addition, investigations of secondary degeneration in the optic nerves of rats, which characterize ongoing changes associated with neurotrauma, have shown that myelin is particularly susceptible to secondary damage.[24,25] Payne and colleagues[25] found a maximum of 15% of myelin sheaths to be decompacted in rats following secondary degeneration. This damage is caused because myelin's compact layers of lamellae are held together with proteins that are vulnerable to damage from reactive oxidative species and lipid peroxidation from secondary degeneration,[26] processes that are known to occur following mTBI.[27,28] Thus, there is circumstantial evidence to support myelin decompaction, a mixture of decompaction and degeneration, and degeneration alone, following mTBI.

Although these findings have been observed in animal models and postmortem human studies, dynamic in vivo studies of myelin damage directly observed in the human brain have been few. A better understanding of myelin damage of humans

in vivo, in the setting of mTBI, could lead to greater insights into the pathophysiology and cognitive/behavioral outcomes, and could greatly improve diagnosis and allow the tracking of brain changes over the recovery period. In addition, it could serve as a marker in therapeutic studies, and may provide novel opportunities for interventional treatments.

IMAGING MYELIN
Diffusion Tensor Imaging

One such attempt at in vivo myelin examination is through diffusion tensor imaging (DTI). DTI is an advanced MR imaging technique that uses magnetic gradients to measure water diffusion in the brain, and, in turn, brain microstructure. This measurement is accomplished by modeling the diffusion data using a symmetric rank-2 positive tensor,[29] which in turn can give information on the amount of diffusion, main direction, and degree of anisotropy. The most commonly reported measures from DTI include mean diffusivity, relative anisotropy, fractional anisotropy (FA), fiber direction maps, and three-dimensional fiber tractography,[30] with FA being the most commonly reported value. Thus, DTI has provided a highly sensitive window into tissue microstructure and changes in white matter, greatly improving understanding of the pathophysiology of mTBI. Although not always in agreement, the most consistently implicated structures affected in mTBI have been the genu of the corpus callosum,[31] the cingulum bundle, the anterior corona radiata, the uncinate fasciculus, and the superior longitudinal fasciculus.[32] Although DTI can detect microstructural changes of white matter that other conventional imaging methods cannot, it lacks the specificity required to identify the parts of the white matter that are being affected, such as the axonal membrane, myelin sheath, or other elements of the microstructure and microarchitecture. For example, Beaulieu and Allen[33] reported in 1994 a similar degree of measured anisotropy in both nonmyelinated olfactory and myelinated trigeminal nerves, showing that myelination is not necessary for diffusional anisotropy. Studies such as these have illustrated the risks of interpreting DTI data as representing white matter changes caused by myelin.[34]

Magnetization Transfer

Another MR imaging method that has been suggested to give insights into changes in myelin is magnetization transfer (MT). MT uses off-resonance excitations to measure magnetization transfer of hydrogen within myelin with surrounding water molecules.[35] In a recently published article in *NMR in Biomedicine*, Lehto and colleagues[36] used the MT ratio using sweep imaging with Fourier transformation (SWIFT) to study potential tissue damage in the thalamocortical pathway in a rat model of TBI, 5 months after injury. They reported decreased MT ratio values, which they suggested indicates mainly demyelination as verified by histologic methods. Although MT represents an exciting technique to measure myelin changes, including a robustness compared with other putative myelin-sensitive techniques, the link between MT and myelin remains unclear. Although several studies support the notion that a change in myelin changes MT,[37–39] it is not necessarily true that a change in MT is caused by a change in myelin. For example, MT can be altered by changes in water content caused by inflammation or edema.[40]

Magnetic Resonance Spectroscopy

In addition, magnetic resonance spectroscopy has been suggested as an option for measuring myelin, given that *N*-acetylaspartate (NAA) has been recently shown to be localized in the oligodendrocytes and myelin of adult rat brains.[41] However, this finding is not specific to myelin, because NAA is also found in neuronal cell bodies and axons.

MYELIN WATER IMAGING

One MR imaging method that does allow specific myelin observations is myelin water imaging (MWI).[42] MWI takes advantage of the fact that the water that exists within the myelin-wrapped bilayers has a short T_2 time of between 10 and 20 milliseconds, whereas intracellular and extracellular water has a T_2 time longer than 60 milliseconds.[43] When measuring T_2 values at various echo times, a resulting T_2 decay curve can be separated into a sum of exponential decays with amplitudes proportional to the relative amounts of water in each domain (**Fig. 1**). From this information, a myelin water fraction (MWF) can be calculated as the ratio of the area of the T_2 distribution arising from myelin water over the area of the entire T_2 distribution, and visually represented as a myelin water image (**Fig. 2**).

MWI has been validated against histopathologic stains in postmortem humans. These studies have shown excellent quantitative correlation between MWF and Luxol fast blue staining (a myelin phospholipid stain) optical density at both 1.5 T and 7 T.[44,45] MWI has also been shown to have high reproducibility in healthy brains, both over time and between imaging sites.[46,47] MWI is the only myelin-specific MR imaging technique to be validated by histopathology, and has provided novel insights into myelin development in normal aging humans, and in demyelination diseases, such as multiple sclerosis (MS).[43] The review by MacKay and Laule[43] provides further details. Recent advances in scanner hardware and pulse sequences have enabled imaging of the whole brain within clinically feasible acquisition times of less than 8 minutes.[48]

Myelin Water Imaging in Mild Traumatic Brain Injuries

To date, only 1 study has used MWI to quantify myelin changes following mTBI damage in human subjects in vivo. Using a repeated-measures design, Wright and colleagues[49] recruited 2 varsity hockey teams (45 players total) and scanned them before the beginning of the athletic competition season.[50] They monitored the players in every game over the season in case of concussive injuries. In the end, 11 players sustained a concussion, and were scanned at 72 hours, 2 weeks, and 2 months postinjury. MR imaging data were acquired on a Philips Achieva 3T scanner using an 8-channel SENSE head coil. Scans included a typical clinical MR imaging work-up (T1-weighted scan, fluid-attenuated inversion recovery [FLAIR], susceptibility-weighted imaging [SWI], DTI), along with a 32-echo T2 scan used to calculate MWF maps (recovery time = 1000 milliseconds; echo times, 10-millisecond intervals from 10 to 320 milliseconds; flip angle = 90°; acquisition matrix = 232 × 192, acquired voxel size 0.99 × 0.99 × 5 mm, reconstructed voxel size = 0.96 × 0.95 × 2.5 mm; time = 14 minutes and 22 seconds). At 2 weeks postinjury, relative to baseline, tract-based spatial statistics revealed significantly reduced MWF in the splenium of the corpus callosum (sCC), left posterior limb of the internal capsule, right posterior thalamic radiation, left superior corona radiata, and left superior longitudinal fasciculus.[49] This finding represented a 5.9% ± 1.2% (mean ± standard error) reduction in MWF from baseline. In the sCC, the reduction was 10% of the baseline value (**Fig. 3**). MWF values at 72 hours and 2 months were not statistically different from baseline, suggesting a greater than 72-hour lag in myelin damage development, and recovery of myelin to preseason levels by around 2 months. However, MWF values at 72 hours did show a reduced trend ($P = .076$). This study leaves open the question as to when peak MWF reduction occurs, because it may take place before or after 2 weeks, and how long it takes for MWF to normalize after injury.

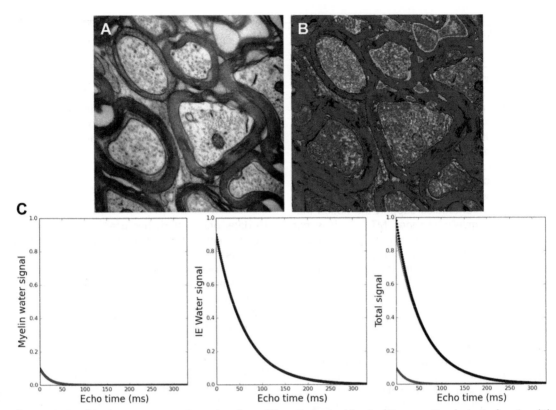

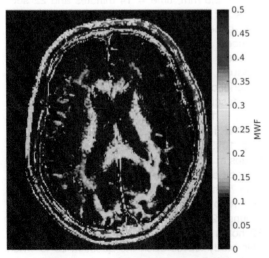

Fig. 1. MWI. White matter cross section taken from C5 cortical spinal tract of Sprague-Dawley rats showing (*A*) myelin sheathes wrapped around axonal tracts, and (*B*) intracellular and extracellular water (*in blue*) and myelin water (*in red*). (*C*) In this simulation, the total signal is assumed to consist of 2 water compartments. One compartment comprises about 10% of the total water within the voxel and has a T2 time of 20 milliseconds (*red decay curve*). The other compartment is 90% of the total water content and its T2 time is 60 milliseconds (*blue curve*). The black curve on the right is the sum of the 2 decay curves. Analyzing a multiecho spin echo MR imaging scan allows the separation of the total multiexponential decay curve into its multiple components. (*Courtesy of [A, B]* Henry Szu-Meng Chen and Piotr Kozlowski, University of British Columbia, Vancouver, British Columbia, Canada.)

Fig. 2. MWF map of a healthy volunteer acquired at 3 T (Philips Ingenia, 32-channel SENSE head coil). (*Courtesy of* Philips Healthcare.)

Cerebrospinal fluid (CSF) serum levels of various proteins in adults and children have been measured after more severe forms of TBI, and concentrations of myelin basic protein in CSF have been found to peak at around 48 to 72 hours.[51] Assuming that the increase in CSF myelin level is coming from myelin breakdown in the brain, Wright and colleagues'[49] findings do not agree with previous literature. However, these studies were performed on more severe types of TBI, suggesting that the mTBI myelin changes that have been observed take longer to occur, and may possibly be different in nature and reversible. Similarly, MWF values may return to baseline sometime after 2 weeks but before 2 months. This study provides the first direct in vivo observation of myelin-specific damage and recovery in humans after a concussion received during contact sports.

Note that although MWI improves imaging specificity for myelin, the technique still does not deliver

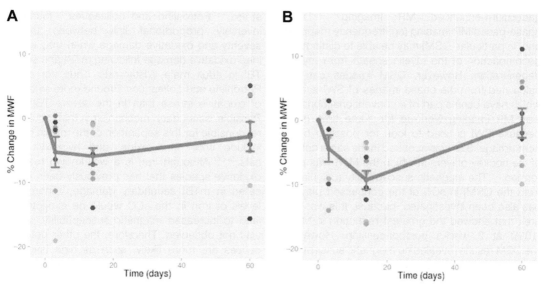

Fig. 3. Relative MWF after concussion. MWF changes relative to baseline, plotted against time for each concussed patient in all significant voxels (*A*) across the whole brain, and (*B*) in the sCC only. Colored data points represent data from each injured athlete (*gray bars* indicate mean ± standard error). Time zero refers to preseason baseline data.

an mTBI signature that clinicians could use to objectively diagnose TBI and TBI severity, as opposed to using self-reported or observed symptoms,[52] which are the equivalent of the Holy Grail in mTBI imaging research. Although MWI does provide a technique that can statistically distinguish brains before and after mTBI at the group level, it cannot equip clinicians with the ability to scan patients after a blast injury, for example, and confidently diagnose them as having (or not having) a TBI, and its level of severity. Such an imaging technique would revolutionize TBI research, treatment, and understanding. Although no such technique yet exists, it is clear that group-level findings can still inform the understanding of TBI and therapeutic practice. For instance, Wright and colleagues'[49] MWI results shed more light on white matter damage that remains despite clinical symptom resolution (a finding also found in various DTI studies; see Eierud and colleagues[31]), thus providing valuable information about when it is safe for someone with a TBI to return to environments that place them in danger of subsequent injuries (eg, in sports or combat).

Limitations

One limitation of MWI is the low signal/noise ratio (SNR) that has so far been achieved, a fact that is hard to mitigate because myelin water makes up approximately 15% of total brain water content.[53] Some ways to increase SNR are to use higher magnetic field strengths, improved receiver

technology, and coils with 32 or more channels. Although greater than 3-T magnets may be too much to ask in a clinical setting, 32-channel head coils and advanced receiver technology are now widely available.

FURTHER INVESTIGATIONS
Quantitative Susceptibility Imaging

Although MWI can produce key insights into the amount and location of myelin changes in vivo, it is not clear from these findings in what way myelin has been altered, because MWF changes can occur because of myelin removal, myelin sheath decompaction, or a mixture of the two.

In order to address this issue, it may be necessary to combine MWI results with another MR imaging technique, such as quantitative susceptibility mapping (QSM). QSM provides a novel contrast mechanism in MR imaging that uses the phase image from gradient echo scans, and computes maps of underlying tissue magnetic susceptibility.[54] Examples of strong modifiers of magnetic susceptibility are paramagnetic (susceptibility greater than zero) iron in deoxygenated blood and the basal ganglia, and diamagnetic (susceptibility less than zero) myelin. In MS, an increase in MR frequency and QSM values has been seen when a reduction in myelin is found during the formation of acute MS lesions.[55–57] This MR frequency technique is highly sensitive, revealing significant changes of up to 3 months before new MS lesions appear on the clinically standard gadolinium-enhanced MR imaging.[55] Thus, phase-based MR imaging (eg, frequency mapping and, in particular, QSM) may be able to distinguish decompaction of the myelin sheath from myelin degeneration. However, QSM images can be calculated from the phase images of SWI scans, which have been a part of a conventional concussion MR imaging work-up for some time now, because SWI is used to look for possible brain hemorrhage. SWI was acquired in the same cohort of ice hockey players in which the MWI was performed.[49] The magnetic susceptibility (calculated from the QSM) in sCC of the concussed players has also been investigated, because this was the area that showed the greatest reduction in MWF (10%) at 2 weeks postconcussion. However, the QSM results revealed no magnetic susceptibility changes at any time point postconcussion (note that these results are tentative because they remain unpublished at the time of writing; however, please refer to Pukropski and colleagues'[58] abstract).

Implications

Can further pathologic insight be found from the joint analysis of MWI and additional scans, such as QSM derived from SWI? Together, the reduction in MWF in the sCC and the absence of changes in magnetic susceptibility in the same region suggests that the myelin sheath structure has been changed through decompaction rather than degeneration.[23,25] Because decompaction leads to a separation of the myelin bilayers, it is expected that T2 relaxation times will increase, reducing the MWF ratio but leaving the local magnetic susceptibility unaffected. This decompaction interpretation is in agreement with the observed recovery of MWF 2 months postinjury, suggesting a normalization of the myelin sheath. Although myelin decompaction may not be as severe an injury as myelin degeneration, there is still reason to view these changes as a serious mTBI disorder, because they lead to reductions in action potential conduction.[59] Myelinated axons in mice and rats have been found to conduct at a rate of 2.4 m/s, which is significantly greater than the unmyelinated rate of 0.4 m/s.[60,61] Axons of mice with decompacted myelin conduct at a rate of about 1.05 m/s.[59] This difference represents a reduction of more than half the conduction rate, and could in turn be responsible for some of the known cognitive deficits following mTBI,[62] such as affected memory, attention, processing speed, and executive functioning. As discussed earlier, myelin decompaction in mTBI is likely to be caused by secondary mechanisms, such as oxidative stress.[25] Petronilho and colleagues[63] found an inversely proportional link between trauma severity and oxidative damage when they examined oxidative damage following mTBI and severe TBI in adult male Wistar rats. Thus, for mTBI, Petronilho and colleagues[63] found more evidence of oxidative stress than in the severe TBI rats. Possible secondary mechanisms that could be responsible for this separation of the myelin layers include iron, nitric oxide, and hydroxyl radicals.[25,28] Although iron is a well-known reactive oxidative species that has previously been implicated in mTBI secondary damage,[28] increased levels of iron in the sCC would be expected to lead to increased magnetic susceptibility, which was not observed. Therefore, the other potential causes are more likely, such as high levels of radical species such as nitric oxide and hydroxyl radicals.[25]

SUMMARY

MWI provides mTBI researchers with a specific myelin biomarker and helps to further elucidate microstructural and microarchitectural changes of white matter after mTBI. Ongoing improvement of scanner hardware and software with the implementation of MWI across scanner platforms will likely result in increased research regarding the role of myelin in TBI. Initial results show altered myelin 2 weeks after concussion and normalization by 2 months after injury. Avenues for future research include a more detailed investigation of myelin between 2 weeks and 2 months after injury, the use of MWI in moderate and severe TBI, and the investigation of the role of myelin in chronic TBI.

REFERENCES

1. Mierzwa AJ, Marion CM, Sullivan GM, et al. Components of myelin damage and repair in the progression of white matter pathology after mild traumatic brain injury. J Neuropathol Exp Neurol 2015;74: 218–32.
2. Armstrong RC, Mierzwa AJ, Marion CM, et al. White matter involvement after TBI: clues to axon and myelin repair capacity. Exp Neurol 2016;275(Pt 3): 328–33.
3. Reeves TM, Phillips LL, Povlishock JT. Myelinated and unmyelinated axons of the corpus callosum differ in vulnerability and functional recovery following traumatic brain injury. Exp Neurol 2005; 196:126–37.
4. Tsunoda I, Fujinami RS. Inside-out versus outside-in models for virus induced demyelination: axonal

damage triggering demyelination. Springer Semin Immunopathol 2002;24:105–25.

5. Shi H, Hu X, Leak RK, et al. Demyelination as a rational therapeutic target for ischemic or traumatic brain injury. Exp Neurol 2015;272:17–25.

6. Smith DH, Meaney DF. Axonal damage in traumatic brain injury. Neuroscientist 2000;6:483–95.

7. Maxwell WL, Bartlett E, Morgan H. Wallerian degeneration in the optic nerve stretch-injury model of traumatic brain injury: a stereological analysis. J Neurotrauma 2015;32:780–90.

8. Christman CW, Grady MS, Walker SA, et al. Ultrastructural studies of diffuse axonal injury in humans. J Neurotrauma 1994;11:173–86.

9. Giza CC, Hovda DA. The neurometabolic cascade of concussion. J Athl Train 2001;36:228–35.

10. Giza CC, Hovda DA. The new neurometabolic cascade of concussion. Neurosurgery 2014; 75(Suppl 4):S24–33.

11. Ellis MJ, Ryner LN, Sobczyk O, et al. Neuroimaging assessment of cerebrovascular reactivity in concussion: current concepts, methodological considerations, and review of the literature. Front Neurol 2016;7:61.

12. Miyamoto N, Maki T, Pham LD, et al. Oxidative stress interferes with white matter renewal after prolonged cerebral hypoperfusion in mice. Stroke 2013;44:3516–21.

13. Flygt J, Djupsjö A, Lenne F, et al. Myelin loss and oligodendrocyte pathology in white matter tracts following traumatic brain injury in the rat. Eur Jm Neurosci 2013;38:2153–65.

14. McCrea M. Mild traumatic brain injury and postconcussion syndrome: the new evidence base for diagnosis and treatment. Oxford (United Kingdom): Oxford University Press; 2007.

15. Benarroch EE. Oligodendrocytes: susceptibility to injury and involvement in neurologic disease. Neurology 2009;72:1779–85.

16. Bailes JE, Dashnaw ML, Petraglia AL, et al. Cumulative effects of repetitive mild traumatic brain injury. Prog Neurol Surg 2014;28:50–62.

17. Ng HK, Mahaliyana RD, Poon WS. The pathological spectrum of diffuse axonal injury in blunt head trauma: assessment with axon and myelin strains. Clin Neurol Neurosurg 1994;96:24–31.

18. Tang-Schomer MD, Johnson VE, Baas PW, et al. Partial interruption of axonal transport due to microtubule breakage accounts for the formation of periodic varicosities after traumatic axonal injury. Exp Neurol 2012;233:364–72.

19. Johnson VE, Stewart JE, Begbie FD, et al. Inflammation and white matter degeneration persist for years after a single traumatic brain injury. Brain 2013;136: 28–42.

20. Liu MC, Akle V, Zheng W, et al. Extensive degradation of myelin basic protein isoforms by calpain following traumatic brain injury. J Neurochem 2006; 98:700–12.

21. Povlishock JT, Katz DI. Update of neuropathology and neurological recovery after traumatic brain injury. J Head Trauma Rehabil 2005;20:76–94.

22. Sullivan GM, Mierzwa AJ, Kijpaisalratana N, et al. Oligodendrocyte lineage and subventricular zone response to traumatic axonal injury in the corpus callosum. J Neuropathol Exp Neurol 2013;72: 1106–25.

23. Donovan V, Kim C, Anugerah AK, et al. Repeated mild traumatic brain injury results in long-term white-matter disruption. J Cereb Blood Flow Metab 2014;34:715–23.

24. Franklin RJM, Ffrench-Constant C. Remyelination in the CNS: from biology to therapy. Nat Rev Neurosci 2008;9:839–55.

25. Payne SC, Bartlett CA, Harvey AR, et al. Myelin sheath decompaction, axon swelling, and functional loss during chronic secondary degeneration in rat optic nerve. Invest Ophthalmol Vis Sci 2012;53: 6093–101.

26. Baumann N, Pham-Dinh D. Biology of oligodendrocyte and myelin in the mammalian central nervous system. Physiol Rev 2001;81:871–927.

27. Kochanek PM, Dixon CE, Shellington DK, et al. Screening of biochemical and molecular mechanisms of secondary injury and repair in the brain after experimental blast-induced traumatic brain injury in rats. J Neurotrauma 2013;30:920–37.

28. Nisenbaum EJ, Novikov DS, Lui YW. The presence and role of iron in mild traumatic brain injury: an imaging perspective. J Neurotrauma 2014;31:301–7.

29. Weickert J, Hagen H. Visualization and processing of tensor fields. New York: Springer Berlin Heidelberg; 2007.

30. Le Bihan D, Mangin JF, Poupon C, et al. Diffusion tensor imaging: concepts and applications. J Magn Reson Imaging 2001;13:534–46.

31. Eierud C, Craddock RC, Fletcher S, et al. Neuroimaging after mild traumatic brain injury: review and meta-analysis. Neuroimage Clin 2014;4: 283–94.

32. Jurick SM, Bangen KJ, Evangelista ND, et al. Advanced neuroimaging to quantify myelin in vivo: application to mild TBI. Brain Inj 2016;30:1452–7.

33. Beaulieu C, Allen PS. Determinants of anisotropic water diffusion in nerves. Magn Reson Med 1994; 31(4):394–400.

34. Beaulieu C. The basis of anisotropic water diffusion in the nervous system - a technical review. NMR Biomed 2002;15:435–55.

35. Stanisz GJ, Kecojevic A, Bronskill MJ, et al. Characterizing white matter with magnetization transfer and T(2). Magn Reson Med 1999;42:1128–36.

36. Lehto LJ, Sierra A, Gröhn O. Magnetization transfer SWIFT MRI consistently detects histologically

verified myelin loss in the thalamocortical pathway after a traumatic brain injury in rat. NMR Biomed 2017;30(2).

37. Schmierer K, Scaravilli F, Altmann DR, et al. Magnetization transfer ratio and myelin in postmortem multiple sclerosis brain. Ann Neurol 2004;56:407–15.

38. Schmierer K, Tozer DJ, Scaravilli F, et al. Quantitative magnetization transfer imaging in postmortem multiple sclerosis brain. J Magn Reson Imaging 2007;26: 41–51.

39. Chen JT, Collins DL, Freedman MS, et al. Local magnetization transfer ratio signal inhomogeneity is related to subsequent change in MTR in lesions and normal-appearing white-matter of multiple sclerosis patients. NeuroImage 2005;25:1272–8.

40. Vavasour IM, Laule C, Li DKB, et al. Is the magnetization transfer ratio a marker for myelin in multiple sclerosis? J Magn Reson Imaging 2011;33:713–8.

41. Nordengen K, Heuser C, Rinholm JE, et al. Localisation of N-acetylaspartate in oligodendrocytes/myelin. Brain Struct Funct 2015;220:899–917.

42. MacKay A, Whittall K, Adler J, et al. In vivo visualization of myelin water in brain by magnetic resonance. Magn Reson Med 1994;31:673–7.

43. MacKay AL, Laule C. Magnetic resonance of myelin water: an in vivo marker for myelin. Brain Plast 2016; 2:71–91.

44. Laule C, Leung E, Lis DK, et al. Myelin water imaging in multiple sclerosis: quantitative correlations with histopathology. Mult Scler 2006;12:747–53.

45. Laule C, Kozlowski P, Leung E, et al. Myelin water imaging of multiple sclerosis at 7 T: correlations with histopathology. NeuroImage 2008;40:1575–80.

46. Meyers SM, Laule C, Vavasour IM, et al. Reproducibility of myelin water fraction analysis: a comparison of region of interest and voxel-based analysis methods. Magn Reson Imaging 2009;27:1096–103.

47. Meyers SM, Vavasour IM, Mädler B, et al. Multicenter measurements of myelin water fraction and geometric mean T2: intra- and intersite reproducibility. J Magn Reson Imaging 2013;38:1445–53.

48. Prasloski T, Rauscher A, MacKay AL, et al. Rapid whole cerebrum myelin water imaging using a 3D GRASE sequence. NeuroImage 2012;63:533–9.

49. Wright AD, Jarrett M, Vavasour I, et al. Myelin water fraction is transiently reduced after a single mild traumatic brain injury - a prospective cohort study in collegiate hockey players. PLoS One 2016;11: e0150215.

50. Jarrett M, Tam R, Hernández-Torres E, et al. A prospective pilot investigation of brain volume, white matter hyperintensities, and hemorrhagic lesions after mild traumatic brain injury. Front Neurol 2016;7:11.

51. Berger RP. The use of serum biomarkers to predict outcome after traumatic brain injury in adults and children. J Head Trauma Rehabil 2006;21:315–33.

52. Blyth BJ, Bazarian JJ. Traumatic alterations in consciousness: traumatic brain injury. Emerg Med Clin North Am 2010;28:571–94.

53. Laule C, Vavasour IM, Kolind SH, et al. Magnetic resonance imaging of myelin. Neurotherapeutics 2007;4:460–84.

54. Schweser F, Deistung A, Lehr BW, et al. Quantitative imaging of intrinsic magnetic tissue properties using MRI signal phase: an approach to in vivo brain iron metabolism? NeuroImage 2011;54:2789–807.

55. Wiggermann V, Hernández Torres E, Vavasour IM, et al. Magnetic resonance frequency shifts during acute MS lesion formation. Neurology 2013;81: 211–8.

56. Wiggermann V, Hametner S, Hernández-Torres E, et al. Susceptibility-sensitive MRI of multiple sclerosis lesions and the impact of normal-appearing white matter changes. NMR Biomed 2017;30(8).

57. Li X, Harrison DM, Liu H, et al. Magnetic susceptibility contrast variations in multiple sclerosis lesions. J Magn Reson Imaging JMRI 2016;43:463–73.

58. Pukropski A, Weber A, Jarrett M, et al. Quantitative susceptibility mapping of hockey players after mild traumatic brain injury. Presented at 25th Annual Meeting and Exhibition of the International Society for Magnetic Resonance in Medicine. Honolulu (HI), April 23–27, 2017.

59. Gutiérrez R, Boison D, Heinemann U, et al. Decompaction of CNS myelin leads to a reduction of the conduction velocity of action potentials in optic nerve. Neurosci Lett 1995;195:93–6.

60. Cahill GM, Menaker M. Responses of the suprachiasmatic nucleus to retinohypothalamic tract volleys in a slice preparation of the mouse hypothalamus. Brain Res 1989;479:65–75.

61. Foster RE, Connors BW, Waxman SG. Rat optic nerve: electrophysiological, pharmacological and anatomical studies during development. Brain Res 1982;255:371–86.

62. Rabinowitz AR, Levin HS. Cognitive sequelae of traumatic brain injury. Psychiatr Clin North Am 2014;37:1–11.

63. Petronilho F, Feier G, de Souza B, et al. Oxidative stress in brain according to traumatic brain injury intensity. J Surg Res 2010;164:316–20.

Susceptibility-Weighted Imaging and Magnetic Resonance Spectroscopy in Concussion

Ivan I. Kirov, PhD[a], Christopher T. Whitlow, MD, PhD, MHA[b,c],
Carlos Zamora, MD, PhD[d,*]

KEYWORDS

- Magnetic resonance spectroscopy (MRS) • Mild traumatic brain injury (mTBI) • Concussion • SWI
- Susceptibility-weighted imaging

KEY POINTS

- Despite its exquisite sensitivity in the detection of intracranial blood products, susceptibility-weighted imaging (SWI) does not play a primary role in mild traumatic brain injury/concussion and its clinical utility is currently limited to assessment of diffuse axonal injury.
- Some studies have shown a correlation between the number, volume, and extent of microhemorrhages on SWI and neurologic outcomes, but results have been mixed.
- The most common proton magnetic resonance spectroscopy (MRS) findings in concussion/mild traumatic brain injury are lower concentrations of N-acetyl-aspartate (indicating compromised neuronal health) and higher levels of choline (indicating glial abnormalities).
- Correlations with clinical outcome, and the property of the spectroscopic markers to show reversible injury, qualifies proton MRS as a potential tool for monitoring recovery from concussion/mild traumatic brain injury.
- Conflicting results caused by study design factors have impeded widespread applications on an individual patient level, and currently proton MRS has most utility in group-level comparisons designed to reveal the pathophysiologic effects of concussion/mild traumatic brain injury.

INTRODUCTION

The prognosis after a traumatic brain injury (TBI) mainly depends on the classifier of mild, moderate, and severe, which is determined by neurologic assessment. In cases in which minimal or no disturbance of consciousness is present, the patient is assigned a score of 15 to 13 on the Glasgow Coma Scale (GCS)[1] and consequently, a designation of mild TBI (mTBI), the most common and least debilitating TBI type. The term concussion has a broader definition, which includes

Disclosure: The authors have nothing to disclose.
[a] Department of Radiology, New York University School of Medicine, Center for Advanced Imaging Innovation and Research (CAI2R), Bernard and Irene Schwartz Center for Biomedical Imaging, 660 First Avenue, 421, New York, NY 10016, USA; [b] Department of Radiology, Division of Neuroradiology, Clinical Translational Sciences Institute, Wake Forest School of Medicine, Medical Center Boulevard, Winston-Salem, NC 27157-8011, USA; [c] Department of Biomedical Engineering, Clinical Translational Sciences Institute, Wake Forest School of Medicine, 1 Medical Center Boulevard, Winston-Salem, NC 27106, USA; [d] Department of Radiology, Division of Neuroradiology, University of North Carolina School of Medicine, University of North Carolina, CB 7510, 3327 Old Infirmary, Chapel Hill, NC 27599-7510, USA
* Corresponding author.
E-mail address: carlos_zamora@med.unc.edu

Neuroimag Clin N Am 28 (2018) 91–105
https://doi.org/10.1016/j.nic.2017.09.007

neuroimaging.theclinics.com

mTBI defined by GCS but also mTBI diagnosed based on retrospective patient report, or based on tools other than the GCS, such as sideline assessment tests used in contact sports.

Despite the overall favorable outcomes after mTBI and concussion (referred to collectively as mTBI henceforth), some patients develop persistent postconcussive symptoms (PCSs) that are not explained by qualitative assessment of conventional MR imaging scans. Given the high incidence of mTBI (>1 million/y in the United States alone),[2] a large body of research has been devoted to developing and testing of techniques sensitive to the subtle MR imaging–occult injury expected in mTBI to address the need for better prognostication through neuroimaging.

Because fractured blood vessels indicate that brain tissue has experienced significant stress/strain, techniques able to detect paramagnetic blood products may be useful for identifying underlying injury.[3,4] One such technique, susceptibility-weighted imaging (SWI), is covered in the first part of this article. SWI is a fully flow-compensated three-dimensional (3D) gradient echo (GRE) sequence that incorporates both magnitude and phase information and that has been shown to be highly sensitive to the signal dephasing caused by paramagnetic blood products (essentially from iron within different states of hemoglobin) and diamagnetic substances (largely calcium).[5] In the setting of moderate and severe TBI, evidence suggests that SWI is significantly more sensitive to hemorrhagic byproducts than its alternative, the T2* GRE sequence.[6] This article reviews the use of SWI in mTBI and discusses its potential added value. Second, it focuses on metabolic imaging by means of magnetic resonance spectroscopy (MRS). Because TBI-associated changes in metabolism can occur even when there are no apparent abnormalities on conventional MR imaging, MRS can provide an additional layer of injury assessment, which, in the case of proton MRS (^{1}H MRS), can be integrated in a standard clinical MR imaging examination. This article therefore reviews the potential clinical utility of ^{1}H MRS, and examines what information its markers have provided about injury mechanisms in mTBI.

PATHOPHYSIOLOGY AND MECHANISMS OF TRAUMATIC BRAIN INJURY

The brain is bathed in cerebrospinal fluid (CSF), which acts like a mechanical cushion and provides a certain degree of motion within the calvarium. During trauma, the brain may be subject to translational, linear, and rotational forces that can generate pressure gradients that result in shearing stress/strain and axonal damage.[7] Depending on the severity of trauma, axonal shearing without intracranial hemorrhage can occur immediately following injury or develop over a longer period of time because of cellular mechanisms that lead to degradation of the cytoskeleton.[8]

Animal Models

Current knowledge of the pathophysiologic mechanisms behind closed head trauma and mTBI are largely derived from animal models that attempt to replicate the injury using low pressure forces. These animal models have generally relied on rodents and with some variations entail the delivery of a force to the intact dura. One of the most extensively used techniques for generating brain trauma in rodent models is via transmission of a fluid pressure pulse (fluid percussion injury).[9] Other techniques involve the use of electromechanically or pneumatically activated rods to deliver a direct force to the brain (controlled cortical impact) or weight drops without the need for a craniectomy.[10]

Neurotransmitter Release, Excitotoxicity, and Ionic Shifts

Cellular distortion with axonal stretching and membrane disruption on impact lead to indiscriminate release of neurotransmitters, efflux of potassium ions, and membrane depolarization.[11] Experimental and clinical studies have shown early release of excitatory neurotransmitters, particularly glutamate, caused by rapid depolarization and also from other potential sources, including extravasation at the site of injury, as well as disruption of the blood-brain barrier.[12] Activation of N-methyl-D-aspartate receptors by glutamate further exacerbates ion transport across the membrane, promoting potassium loss and influx of calcium ions, as well as further membrane depolarization.[13] Intracellular accumulation of calcium results in activation of calcium-dependent proteases, mitochondrial dysfunction, and release of oxygen free radicals adding to cellular injury.[8,10,11] Activity of the Na^+/K^+ ATPase pump increases in an attempt to restore the transmembrane ion gradients. The resultant increased glucose metabolism is exacerbated by mitochondrial dysfunction and promotes anaerobic metabolism with increased accumulation of lactate and local acidosis.[14] A second stage of postimpact injury is thought to involve hypometabolism, hypoperfusion, and further disruption of the blood-brain barrier with ensuing edema.[15] However, some data in patients with mTBI suggest that, at least in the acute setting, there may be increases in cerebral blood flow to certain areas of the brain.[16]

Neuroinflammation

Release of intracellular products and generation of free radicals during TBI is characterized by a prominent neuroinflammatory response that involves activation of quiescent microglia within hours in a process known as reactive gliosis.[10,17] Whether cells are activated in response to secondary factors, or are primarily pathogenic, is not clear.[18] Local activation of microglia leads to release of oxygen free radicals, cytokines (eg, interleukin-1β, tumor necrosis factor-α, and transforming growth factor-1β), and proteases that perpetuate the inflammatory response, as well as recruitment of peripheral immune cells through a permeable blood-brain barrier, including neutrophils, macrophages, and lymphocytes.[10,19] The inflammatory cascade elicited by trauma and other injuries can have lasting effects over the following weeks, months, and years, and possibly promotes neurodegeneration over time, although whether it also plays a role in neural repair is uncertain.[18]

SUSCEPTIBILITY-WEIGHTED IMAGING
Technical Aspects

Principles

Magnetic susceptibility is the magnetic behavior of a substance when it is placed under an external magnetic field. This property allows SWI to characterize tissues with different magnetic susceptibilities that may otherwise be difficult to discriminate with conventional MR imaging techniques. Although phase data acquired during MR imaging scanning contain a large amount of tissular susceptibility information, these were typically discarded in the past with the exception of certain vascular or flow applications. Phase information is now exploited to generate SWI sequences with very high sensitivity for the detection of paramagnetic and diamagnetic substances in the brain.

Merging of phase and magnitude

The basic process in the generation of SWI starts with the separate acquisition of magnitude and phase data. Phase images are rich in susceptibility information from the interrogated tissues, and tissue-associated differences can be enhanced by the use of sufficiently long echo times and are more pronounced at larger magnetic field strengths.[20] However, phase sequences also include many unwanted artifacts from magnetic field inhomogeneities, which are greatest at air-tissue interfaces, most notably those that occur between the osseous structures of the skull base and paranasal sinuses, as well as the adjacent cerebral parenchyma and pituitary gland. These artifacts profoundly obscure the structures of interest and limit evaluation of raw phase images, but, because they tend to occur at low frequencies, they can be removed by the application of a high-pass filter.

After the raw phase images have been filtered, a phase mask is created by suppressing pixels with certain phase values thus enhancing contrast, the result of which is then multiplied by the magnitude images to produce the final SWI sequence.[5] This sequence can be further postprocessed to create thick minimum-intensity projections (minIPs) that increase the conspicuity of small lesions by staying longer in the observer's field of view while scrolling through a data set (Fig. 1). By combining magnitude and phase information, SWI is able to display the high resolution and T2 contrast effects from the former, and the susceptibility information from the latter, in a single sequence.[5] Generation of SWI images can be achieved in as short a time as 4 to 5 minutes.

Detection of paramagnetic and diamagnetic substances

SWI has gained popularity largely because of its exquisite sensitivity for the detection of paramagnetic substances that exert local susceptibility effects and result in signal dephasing. Most applications are related to iron within different states of hemoglobin, in which the degree of paramagnetism depends primarily on the number of unpaired electrons in the molecule.[21] The oxyhemoglobin in hyperacute hemorrhage has no unpaired electrons and therefore is only weakly diamagnetic and does not result in significant dephasing on SWI. Deoxyhemoglobin is formed when the heme moieties lose their oxygen molecules, allowing 4 unpaired electrons and resulting in a strong paramagnetic effect. Therefore, deoxyhemoglobin in acute hematomas and in deoxygenated blood produces significant signal loss on SWI.[20] Deoxyhemoglobin subsequently undergoes oxidation to methemoglobin, which has an additional unpaired electron that makes it even more paramagnetic and even more conspicuous on SWI.[22]

The susceptibility effects of diamagnetic substances are not as strong as those of paramagnetic ones, but are nonetheless significant enough to produce signal dephasing on SWI. For imaging purposes, calcium is the most important diamagnetic substance in the human body, where it occurs mostly in the form of calcium phosphates.

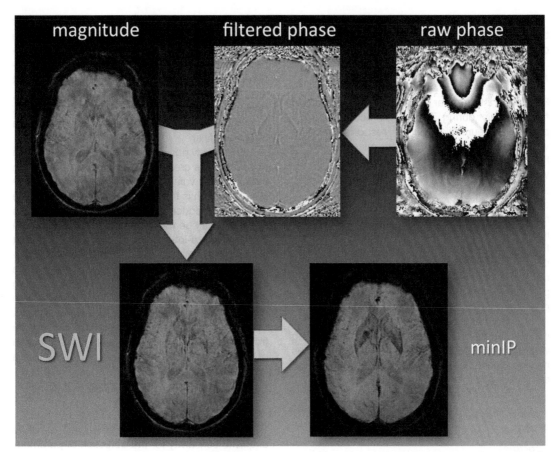

Fig. 1. Key steps in the generation of an SWI sequence. Major artifacts from the phase data set in the upper right image are seen predominantly anteriorly because of air-tissue interfaces at the paranasal sinuses. These low-frequency variations are eliminated after a high-pass filter. After creating a phase mask, the filtered phase images are combined with the magnitude data creating the SWI sequence. A 15-mm minIP in the lower right image helps to increase lesion conspicuity.

Susceptibility-Weighted Imaging in Traumatic Brain Injury

Overview

Computed tomography (CT) continues to be the mainstay in the management of acute TBI.[23] However, in the absence of specific clinical findings (headache, vomiting, substance intoxication, deficits in short-term memory, physical evidence of trauma above the clavicles, or seizure), patients who are less than 60 years of age and who present with minor head trauma can sometimes be safely discharged without the need for head CT or other neuroimaging.[24]

Indications for performing MR imaging in the acute or subacute settings are not as well established and tend to vary by institution. The American College of Radiology Head Injury Institute does not recommend performance of MR imaging in acute brain trauma because of the logistics involved and resource availability, except

when noncontrast head CT is normal and there are persistent unexplained neurologic deficits (class I recommendation).[4] The major potential role of SWI in acute trauma revolves around its superb ability to detect blood products. It is well established that SWI has significantly increased sensitivity for microhemorrhages and improved visualization of hemorrhagic volume load compared with CT and other MR imaging techniques (**Fig. 2**).[6,25–28] However, differences in hemorrhage detection between SWI and other MR imaging sequences may only be evident with small hemorrhages, and whether there is a clinical or prognostic benefit from detecting a larger number of them in trauma is inconclusive. In diffuse axonal injury (DAI), Tao and colleagues[29] in 2015 showed that SWI was better able to detect hemorrhagic foci compared with other MR imaging sequences, including conventional gradient echo, but this difference was only significant for hemorrhages that were 10 mm or less in diameter.

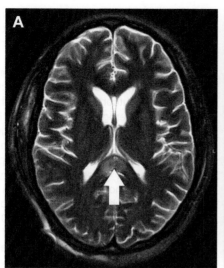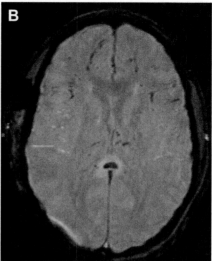

Fig. 2. The increased sensitivity of SWI for hemorrhage is shown in this patient with diffuse axonal injury (DAI). Axial T2-weighted image (*A*) shows focal hyperintensity in the splenium of the corpus callosum with a hypointense center (*arrow*) but no other major abnormality. Minimum-intensity SWI projection (*B*) shows the focal splenial hemorrhage to better advantage and also outlines thalamic lesions and extensive white matter shear injury, which appears as linear hypointensities in the anterior cerebrum.

Number and volume of microhemorrhages

Several studies have used SWI to evaluate the presence of microhemorrhages in mTBI, but results have been inconsistent, and currently SWI does not play a primary role in diagnosis. Although some studies have reported an increased number of microhemorrhages in patients with mTBI,[30] most have shown no significant differences, and SWI is frequently normal in studies that have included a control population.[31–36] A study of concussed hockey players published in 2016 did not show any signs of injury on SWI even at 3.0 T and using a multiecho technique with improved signal/noise and contrast/noise ratios.[32,37] In a recent study by Trifan and colleagues,[30] the prevalence of hemorrhages in SWI in patients with mTBI was 17%, which included microhemorrhages, contusions, and extra-axial hemorrhage, and their detection increased proportionately with the severity of TBI. In the pediatric population, a study by Maugans and colleagues[31] that included 12 children who had experienced a single sports-related concussion did not show microhemorrhages or any other abnormalities on SWI or anatomic MR imaging sequences. The number of subjects in most of these studies has been small and therefore findings are not conclusive.

A larger study by Huang and colleagues[38] investigated the prevalence of microhemorrhages in a cohort of 111 patients with mTBI compared with controls. Microhemorrhages were 4 times more common in the mTBI group and were frequently located at the gray matter (GM)–white matter (WM) junction.[38] However, the study included a wide range of ages and did not control for other potential age-related causes for the microhemorrhages, and therefore attributing these microhemorrhages to trauma with any degree of certainty is difficult.[38] In a separate study, Wang and colleagues[39] found a microhemorrhage prevalence of 19.4% in 165 subjects 1 year after mTBI; however, they lacked a noninjured control group for comparison.

Contact sports

There has been particular interest in contact sports given the potential for repetitive concussive injuries and subconcussive exposures. SWI was used as part of the neuroradiological, clinical, and neuropsychological evaluation of 45 retired National Football League (NFL) players (sponsored by the NFL), in which the number of microhemorrhages was associated with the number of football impacts reported for an individual but not with the total number of concussions. However, the study was limited by the lack of a true control group and the fact that, of the 4 subjects with microhemorrhages, 1 had a history of severe TBI that likely accounted for the SWI abnormalities.[40] A separate study comparing amateur boxers with control subjects did find more microhemorrhages in the boxers, but the difference was not statistically significant.[33]

Measurement of hypointensity burden

Although many studies have concentrated on measuring the number and volume of lesions, Helmer and colleagues[41] used a different approach in their study of ice hockey players published in 2014. Citing neuropathologic studies that showed submillimeter pericapillary hemosiderin staining and claiming that such changes may be too small to detect on visual inspection of SWI, they used an automated method to measure the entire SWI hypointensity burden in the brain (after removal of venous structures) and found that this metric significantly increased throughout the course of the season and particularly in male subjects.

Susceptibility-weighted imaging and mapping

Haacke and colleagues[42] developed a variation of the SWI technique whereby a regularized inverse filter is applied to the frequency domain of the phase data creating susceptibility maps that are unaffected by the orientation of the vessels and that allow quantification and visualization of venous blood. Using this technique, they showed increased oxygenation in areas of increased regional perfusion (measured by arterial spin labeling) in acute mTBI, specifically in the left striatum, frontal lobes, and parietal lobes, compared with controls.[16] Increased perfusion to these areas results in decreased cerebral extraction fraction and a decreased content of deoxyhemoglobin in venous blood, which diminishes the intensity of signal dephasing. However, the high susceptibility of SWI to changes in venous oxygen saturation and ventilation status[43] is likely to introduce measurement variability and therefore the utility of this technique remains to be determined.

Susceptibility-weighted imaging and prediction of neurologic outcomes

Studies of SWI in patients who were clinically diagnosed with DAI have shown a strong correlation between the number of microhemorrhages and GCS.[29,44] In their evaluation of 40 children with DAI, Tong and colleagues[44] also found that the number of microhemorrhages were predictive of neurologic outcomes: those subjects who experienced only mild disability or a normal outcome had on average fewer and a smaller volume of lesions compared with those with moderate to severe disability at 6 to 12 months after injury. In a separate evaluation of 18 children with different severities of trauma, lesion volume, and to a lesser extent lesion number, were negatively correlated with neuropsychological outcomes and intelligence quotient 1 to 4 years after injury.[22] Another SWI study in 40 children with TBI showed a significant difference in lesion extension between

normal/mild outcome and poor outcome groups 6 to 12 months after injury using the Pediatric Cerebral Performance Category Scale score.[36] However, in a different cohort of patients including mild, moderate, and severe TBI, Chastain and colleagues[45] did not find SWI to be predictive using the Glasgow Outcome Scale score, although the data were heterogeneous and the length of follow-up was widely variable. In patients with only mTBI, Huang and colleagues[38] noted that those who had microhemorrhages performed more poorly in short-term memory testing compared with those without, although comparisons against or within the control group were not performed. In another study of 200 patients with mTBI, the number and volume of microhemorrhages detected on SWI were greater in patients who developed depression after trauma compared with those who did not.[39]

MAGNETIC RESONANCE SPECTROSCOPY
Technical Aspects

Overview

The basis of MRS is the chemical shift effect, which describes the property of a nucleus of the same element to resonate at different frequencies depending on the chemical bonds of the molecule in which it is located. Another way to characterize this principle is that different molecules can be distinguished based on the frequencies at which their nuclei resonate. The main value of MRS in radiology comes from quantifying the resonating hydrogen (proton, ^1H) nuclei, and, by inference, the amount of their parent molecules. ^1H MRS is unique among metabolic imaging techniques in that it is available on all major commercial MR scanners, allowing neurochemical information to be seamlessly integrated with the neuroanatomy provided by the ubiquitous T1-weighted and T2-weighted imaging. In total, ^1H MRS can detect more than a dozen metabolites in neural tissue, but most are hard to quantify and require ultra high magnetic field strength or dedicated acquisition protocols and postprocessing approaches. At clinical magnet strength (≤ 3 T) the main quantifiable metabolites in the brain are N-acetyl-aspartate (NAA), creatine (Cr), choline (Cho), myo-inositol (mI), and the sum of glutamate (Glu) and glutamine (Gln), known as Glx (Fig. 3). Less common are studies performing independent measurements of Glu and Gln, as well as of other harder to measure metabolites such as gamma-aminobutyric acid (GABA). The concentrations of all these metabolites, as measured by ^1H MRS, can be affected in disease, with the directionality of the change (increase or decrease) reflecting

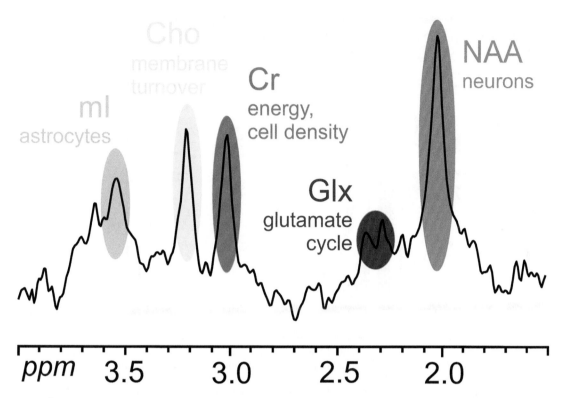

Fig. 3. ^{1}H MRS, short echo time, brain in vivo spectrum showing the major resonances in healthy tissue and their general specificities.

different aspects of cellular health. Such information can be obtained from individual regions on the scale of few cubic centimeters, or over large parts of the brain. These and other considerations of ^{1}H MRS are expanded on later and the results of applications in mTBI are summarized.

[1]H magnetic resonance spectroscopy approaches

Even though ^{1}H MRS sequences exist in a large number of incarnations, users choose between 2 general ^{1}H MRS moieties: single voxel and multivoxel. The more widespread version is single-voxel ^{1}H MRS, in which a spectrum is obtained from a volume of approximately 2 to 8 cm^3, which can be tailored in a cube or cuboid shape depending on the brain area in which it is placed. The single-voxel approach has 2 welcome attributes for clinical use: its short acquisition time and high metabolite signal/noise ratio (SNR). Depending on the application, these are weighed against drawbacks such as the inability to study a large number of regions in the same session and possible voxel contamination with unwanted tissue in the large (on the scale of the brain) single-voxel volume. To probe more tissue, two-dimensional or 3D spectral matrices can

be acquired using multivoxel ^{1}H MRS (eg, Fig. 4), which is a term used interchangeably with chemical shift imaging and ^{1}H MR spectroscopic imaging. The large coverage with a typical spatial resolution (voxel size) of approximately 1 cm^3 allows the testing of a wide range of hypotheses, including those generated retrospectively about regions not thought to be implicated at scanning time. However, the smaller voxel size compared with single-voxel ^{1}H MRS results in lower SNR, which needs to be made up in longer acquisitions and averaging across multiple voxels in order to obtain more reproducible data.

[1]H magnetic resonance spectroscopy acquisition

In addition to high SNR, narrow metabolite linewidth is also critical to spectral quality. Variations in the homogeneity of the main magnetic field within the ^{1}H MRS region give rise to broadened linewidths that decrease the spectral resolution and thereby the fidelity of quantification. To avoid this pitfall, a key aspect preceding any ^{1}H MRS acquisition is shimming, which changes the currents in a set of dedicated coils to achieve as much magnetic homogeneity as possible. After

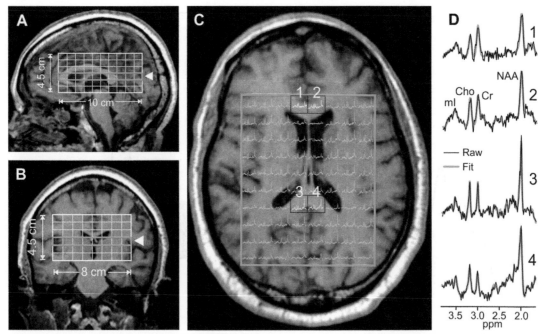

Fig. 4. Sagittal (*A*) and coronal (*B*) T1-weighted MR imaging of a patient with mTBI, showing the placement of a multivoxel ¹H MRS volume of interest, containing 6 spectroscopic slices. The 8 × 10-cm spectral matrix from the slice outlined in blue and indicated by the arrowheads is shown in (*C*), overlaid on a corresponding T1-weighted axial image. The voxel size is 0.75 cm³. Spectra from the corpus callosum are outlined and shown in white, with *1* and *2* originating from the genu, and *3* and *4* from the splenium. They are magnified in (*D*) with their fitted model functions (*gray lines*) used for estimating the metabolite areas. The corpus callosum is vulnerable to TBI (see **Fig. 2**) and is therefore frequently studied with ¹H MRS. This patient, with no findings on conventional MR imaging, was part of a group-level analysis of global (over the entire volume of interest) metabolite concentrations, which found lower white matter NAA levels in patients compared with controls. (*Data from* Kirov II, Tal A, Babb JS, et al. Diffuse axonal injury in mild traumatic brain injury: a 3D multivoxel proton MR spectroscopy study. J Neurol 2013;260(1):242–52.)

shimming and adjustment of other parameters such as water suppression, the single-voxel or multivoxel experiment is performed using any of several localization paradigms, the most common of which is point-resolved spectroscopy.[46]

¹H magnetic resonance spectroscopy postprocessing and quantification

Depending on the sequence and the nature of the experiment, the postprocessing ranges from full automation at the scanner console (eg, for sequences provided by the MR scanner vendor) to being highly dependent on user input (eg, for custom sequences and software). A key step in all pipelines is quantifying the peak areas to assess deviations from normal metabolism. Although line fitting performed by on-scanner software is sufficient for aiding radiological assessment of spectra in clinical cases, more rigorous quantification is advised in research applications. Several software packages available for offline use offer more sophisticated fitting approaches, coupled with tools for automatic spectral quality control. These

results can be coregistered with GM, WM, and CSF masks segmented from structural MR imaging to account for partial volume effects.

¹H MRS results are expressed either as metabolic ratios (eg, NAA/Cr), institutional units, or biochemical units (eg, millimoles per kilogram of wet weight). Ratios are widely used because they are easy to derive, account for several instrumental factors, and results can be compared with published cutoffs designating an abnormal result.[47] However, when the metabolic changes are subtle, it cannot be ascertained whether changes in the ratio are caused by the numerator, denominator, or both. Quantification in institutional or biochemical units with the appropriate corrections and referencing steps provides unambiguous interpretation of the results but is more time consuming and error prone.[48] The appropriate quantification method for a given study can be chosen based on estimation of the population means and standard deviations of the intended numerator and denominator.[49]

Major ^{1}H magnetic resonance spectroscopy metabolites

N-acetyl-aspartate NAA is an amino-acid derivative synthesized in the mitochondria and found exclusively in the cell bodies, dendrites, and axons of neurons.[50] Although its precise role is unclear, studies correlating NAA changes with neuronal density, cytoarchitecture, metabolism, and function[51,52] have established the metabolite as a marker of neurons.

Creatine The ^{1}H MRS Cr peak is more constant and invariant compared to the other metabolites,[53] motivating the NAA/Cr ratio, which is a commonly used metric to infer NAA levels.[54] However, the Cr concentration can also be independently interpreted as a marker of cellular density and energy metabolism.[55,56]

Choline Cho levels are interpreted as a measure of the combined rates of membrane synthesis and degradation. Either of those two events would therefore result in increase of the Cho signal. In the brain, this occurs in the context of most neoplasms, gliosis, and demyelination/remyelination.

Myo-inositol The mI resonance is only visible at short echo times because of its fast signal decay caused by J-coupled dephasing. ^{1}H MRS-detected mI has been shown to originate from a single cell type, the astrocyte.[57] Consequently, mI levels may indicate glial status, with a relationship having been established with astrogliosis.[58]

Glutamate and glutamine Because of the proximity of their major resonances around 2.4 ppm (see **Fig. 3**), Glu and Gln are usually not reliably distinguished at clinical magnetic field strengths ($\leq$3 T).[59] However, their sum, referred to as Glx,[59] can be quantified with high accuracy even at 0.5 T with standard sequences,[60] underlining the fact that measurement of Glx is directly translatable for clinical use.

^{1}H Magnetic Resonance Spectroscopy in Mild Traumatic Brain Injury

Overview

Since the first application in mTBI 20 years ago,[61] the sensitivity of ^{1}H MRS to TBI-inflicted injury in normal-appearing tissue has been well established. ^{1}H MRS abnormalities have been reported in numerous GM and WM regions with both single-voxel and multivoxel methodologies. Commonly studied are, for GM, the cingulate gyrus,[62–64] dorsolateral prefrontal cortex,[65–67] and deep GM,[63,64,68,69] and, for WM, frontal[31,70–73] and supraventricular[56,63,69,74–76] regions, as well as splenium[56,61,77,78] and genu[77,78] of the corpus callosum (eg, see **Fig. 4**). The multifocal nature of TBI damage also lends itself to global ^{1}H MRS approaches,[56,76,79,80] with most methods using multivoxel data to yield 1 metabolic concentration per tissue type over a large brain area ($\sim$80–300 cm^3).

The primary findings are lower NAA[64,65,71,72,77,78,80,81] and higher Cho levels,[62,82,83] assessed either in absolute amounts or ratios. The magnitude of these abnormalities increases with injury severity, as assessed by GCS,[84] neuropsychological test scores,[82] duration of posttraumatic amnesia,[84] and MR imaging findings.[85] Secondary findings are increased mI,[68,83] whereas the data are less consistent for Cr and Glx. There is evidence for both higher[56,74] and lower[86] Cr levels, with a recent study suggesting that, in more severe TBI, these findings are not mutually exclusive.[82] The Glx literature is also split; for example, both higher[62,68] and lower levels[56,74] have been reported in GM. These findings are in contrast with more severe TBI, in which Glx is invariably found to be higher.[87,88]

Of note, there are results that do not correspond with the wide trends. Examples include lower Cho/Cr[69] and mI/Cr,[89] as well as many instances of null findings,[63,90] including in a rare mTBI study in pediatrics.[31] The discrepancies are likely caused by differences in the studied tissue (GM/WM), region, ^{1}H MRS technique, and postprocessing, as well as TBI stage, type, and patient population.

Contact sports

Most MRS studies of the general population exclude patients with previous mTBI because of concern for cumulative injury, which can lead to different pathophysiology and recovery mechanisms. These aspects of mTBI are the subject of study in athletes of contact sports. The 2 main areas of interest in this population are related to contributing to return-to-play guidelines and to understanding the long-term effects of repetitive mTBI.

The acute period after sports mTBI has been associated with metabolic abnormalities of the type seen in other mTBI (eg, lower NAA/Cr), both in GM[65] and WM.[71,73] Concussion history before the studied mTBI seems to matter: one study found that the first clinically diagnosed mTBI event was associated with the greatest reduction of NAA/Cr and NAA/Cho ratios, suggesting that metabolic response depends on the number of previous mTBIs. During the subacute stage, metabolism may normalize over time,[71,73] but a second mTBI event within a vulnerable period of approximately 30 days was shown to result in a WM NAA/Cr deficit that resolved slower than after a single mTBI.[73] The notion of eventual full metabolic recovery is supported by one study examining the long-term effects of mTBI, which found no differences at 1 year.[91] However, the same region studied in a different cohort at 6 months produced metabolite-dependent findings: some abnormalities resolved, whereas others did not.[92]

For a meaningful interpretation of the results in different studies, the effect of repetitive mTBI needs to be taken into account. One longitudinal study showed that metabolic changes can occur over time without association with a particular mTBI event: in a cohort of actively competing martial arts fighters, not recruited after a concussion but with a history or multiple mTBI, WM NAA declined over 1 year. A cross-sectional study on the long-term effects of repetitive mTBI found higher GM Cho and Glx in retired professional athletes (also without recent mTBI).[62]

Another important consideration is the potential effect of head impacts that do not result in an mTBI diagnosis. There is now diffusion tensor imaging[93] and ^{1}H MRS evidence that such so-called subconcussions result in microstructural[93] and metabolic (higher GM Cho and mI levels)[83] abnormalities. Whether there is clinical significance to these findings is yet to be determined, but, for purposes of study design, subconcussions may need to be accounted for, especially in cases in which the control group consists of contact sports athletes.

[1]H magnetic resonance spectroscopy and prediction of neurologic outcomes

The spectroscopic markers have shown prognostic utility: consistent findings in moderate/severe TBI show that lower NAA/Cr[94–99] and higher Cho/Cr[88,97] ratios are related to poor long-term clinical outcome. Serial follow-up allowing comparison between changes in metabolism and in clinical state show that those patients who do not recover have lesser mean increases in NAA/Cr ratio over the follow-up period.[97,100,101] These findings are supported by nonimaging studies: cerebral microdialysis showed that poor outcome was observed only in patients whose extracellular NAA failed to recover,[102] and liquid chromatography NAA levels in an animal model were reduced proportionally to injury severity, with recovery to normal levels only in the less injured group.[103]

Although the prognostic data discussed earlier are from more severe TBI, there is evidence that ^{1}H MRS is also associated with outcome in mTBI. Findings related to self-reported PCS include higher GM Cho/Cr ratio in patients with sensory symptoms, compared with those without[64]; lower global WM NAA level in patients with at least 1 PCS at the time of scanning, but normal metabolism in PCS-free patients[104];

correlation between lower GM NAA/Cr and Glu/Cr ratios and symptom severity[65]; and no ^{1}H MRS differences between controls and an asymptomatic mTBI cohort.[91] Statistical trends were found between PCS and WM Glx,[74] and for lower WM NAA/Cr ratio in patients with chronic versus resolved headache.[75] Although serial studies have shown that symptoms can resolve as metabolism returns to normal levels,[71,73] the timing does not necessarily coincide, because lower WM NAA/Cr ratio can persist despite the lack of PCS.[71,78]

Fewer studies have performed neuropsychological testing, with some reporting no relationship with ^{1}H MRS,[74,78] and others finding correlations with WM Cr[56,69] and NAA levels.[72]

However, no conflicting data are present in the literature of studies specifically recruiting subjects sharing common chronic PCS symptoms. Compared with controls, patients with memory impairment showed lower NAA/Cr and NAA/Cho ratios in the hippocampus,[81] and those with headache showed lower WM NAA/Cr and higher WM Cho/Cr ratios.[75] In a mild to moderate TBI cohort, the presence of pain and its severity were both associated with lower NAA/Cr ratio in the insula.[105]

In addition, 1 study divided the patients into 2 groups, 1 with confirmed loss of consciousness and 1 without, and found that the former had lower NAA levels in the brainstem.[72]

Data interpretation

A single observation of low NAA is not informative of cause (ie, neuronal loss or dysfunction), but serial studies reporting normalization of levels[71,73,106] suggest that a large component of the NAA signal is representative of function. Therefore, NAA is an excellent candidate for monitoring disorders such as mTBI because of its property to dynamically reflect neuronal viability and track reversible damage.[107] The strongest evidence for a biological correlate of these changes supports a link to mitochondrial function.[108,109]

Signal changes in Cho and Cr levels can each be interpreted differently depending on the timing of the scan. In acute TBI, higher Cho levels may indicate damage to cell membranes/myelin and higher Cr levels may reflect energy disbalance.[56] However, in chronic TBI, these abnormalities may be caused by gliosis,[55] an interpretation that can be corroborated by concurrent increase of mI level.

Although it can be postulated that excitotoxicity is related to higher Glx, this remains speculative because of the lack of knowledge of how the Glx signal reflects changes in the glutamate cycle.

SUMMARY

Numerous studies have established that SWI is significantly more sensitive than other imaging modalities in the detection of intracranial blood products. Although some studies of patients with mTBI have suggested an increased incidence of microhemorrhages on SWI, most have been unable to show a significant difference compared with controls and the clinical role of SWI in TBI has been primarily limited to the assessment of DAI. Some studies have shown a potential role in the prediction of neurologic outcomes according to the number of microhemorrhages and lesion extension; however, results have been mixed, possibly because of the varied methodologies and small numbers of subjects. Inherent drawbacks in evaluating the presence of microhemorrhages include the inability to time these lesions from a single scan and the difficulty in attributing microhemorrhages to a specific concussive event unless there is unequivocal documentation with pretraumatic and posttraumatic scans. In older patients, other causes of spontaneous microhemorrhage must be accounted for, particularly amyloid angiopathy, which can show a similar pattern of peripheral distribution to that described in some patients with TBI. Consequently, the isolated presence of microhemorrhages is not by itself contributory in an individual with mTBI. A preliminary quantitative study has shown the potential utility of SWI in evaluating the entire cerebral hypointensity burden, which could, at least theoretically, detect microhemorrhages that may be too small to identify by visual inspection, although such results need to be validated. A different approach includes quantification of susceptibility changes in venous blood as a surrogate for perfusion, although some variability is expected to be caused by ventilation status and oxygen saturation.

With regard to ^{1}H MRS, a large body of literature has established the presence of metabolic abnormalities in normal-appearing tissue of patients with mTBI. The main findings are lower NAA and higher Cho levels, expressed in absolute amounts or in metabolic ratios. In line with the diffuse nature of TBI, these and other abnormalities have been found in regions throughout the brain. Correlations with clinical outcome, and the property of the spectroscopic markers to show reversible injury, qualifies ^{1}H MRS as a potential tool for monitoring recovery from mTBI. However, conflicting results caused by study design factors have impeded widespread applications on an individual patient level, and currently ^{1}H MRS has most utility in group-level comparisons designed to reveal the pathophysiologic effects of mTBI.

REFERENCES

1. Teasdale G, Jennett B. Assessment of coma and impaired consciousness. A practical scale. Lancet 1974;2(7872):81–4.
2. Faul M, Xu L, Wald MM, et al. Traumatic Brain Injury in the United States: Emergency Department Visits, Hospitalizations and Deaths 2002–2006. Atlanta (GA): Centers for Disease Control and Prevention, National Center for Injury Prevention and Control; 2010.
3. Wintermark M, Coombs L, Druzgal TJ, et al. Traumatic brain injury imaging research roadmap. AJNR Am J Neuroradiol 2015;36(3):E12–23.
4. Wintermark M, Sanelli PC, Anzai Y, et al. Imaging evidence and recommendations for traumatic brain injury: conventional neuroimaging techniques. J Am Coll Radiol 2015;12(2):e1–14.
5. Haacke EM, Mittal S, Wu Z, et al. Susceptibility-weighted imaging: technical aspects and clinical applications, part 1. AJNR Am J Neuroradiol 2009;30(1):19–30.
6. Tong KA, Ashwal S, Holshouser BA, et al. Hemorrhagic shearing lesions in children and adolescents with posttraumatic diffuse axonal injury: improved detection and initial results. Radiology 2003;227(2):332–9.
7. Blennow K, Brody DL, Kochanek PM, et al. Traumatic brain injuries. Nat Rev Dis Primers 2016;2: 16084.
8. Shin SS, Bales JW, Edward Dixon C, et al. Structural imaging of mild traumatic brain injury may not be enough: overview of functional and metabolic imaging of mild traumatic brain injury. Brain Imaging Behav 2017;11(2):591–610.
9. Lyeth BG. Historical review of the fluid-percussion TBI model. Front Neurol 2016;7:217.
10. Choe MC. The pathophysiology of concussion. Curr Pain Headache Rep 2016;20(6):42.
11. Giza CC, Hovda DA. The neurometabolic cascade of concussion. J Athl Train 2001;36(3):228–35.
12. Yi JH, Hazell AS. Excitotoxic mechanisms and the role of astrocytic glutamate transporters in traumatic brain injury. Neurochem Int 2006;48(5):394–403.
13. Blanke ML, VanDongen AMJ, Chapter 13. Activation Mechanisms of the NMDA Receptor. In: VanDongen AM, editor. Biology of the NMDA Receptor. Boca Raton (FL): CRC Press/Taylor & Francis; 2009.
14. Barkhoudarian G, Hovda DA, Giza CC. The molecular pathophysiology of concussive brain injury - an update. Phys Med Rehabil Clin N Am 2016;27(2): 373–93.
15. Dashnaw ML, Petraglia AL, Bailes JE. An overview of the basic science of concussion and subconcussion: where we are and where we are going. Neurosurg Focus 2012;33(6):E5: 1-9.

16. Doshi H, Wiseman N, Liu J, et al. Cerebral hemodynamic changes of mild traumatic brain injury at the acute stage. PLoS One 2015;10(2):e0118061.

17. Burda JE, Sofroniew MV. Reactive gliosis and the multicellular response to CNS damage and disease. Neuron 2014;81(2):229–48.

18. Russo MV, McGavern DB. Inflammatory neuroprotection following traumatic brain injury. Science 2016;353(6301):783–5.

19. Chiu CC, Liao YE, Yang LY, et al. Neuroinflammation in animal models of traumatic brain injury. J Neurosci Methods 2016;272:38–49.

20. Ong BC, Stuckey SL. Susceptibility weighted imaging: a pictorial review. J Med Imaging Radiat Oncol 2010;54(5):435–49.

21. Bradley WG Jr. MR appearance of hemorrhage in the brain. Radiology 1993;189(1):15–26.

22. Thomas B, Somasundaram S, Thamburaj K, et al. Clinical applications of susceptibility weighted MR imaging of the brain - a pictorial review. Neuroradiology 2008;50(2):105–16.

23. Joseph B, Friese RS, Sadoun M, et al. The BIG (brain injury guidelines) project: defining the management of traumatic brain injury by acute care surgeons. J Trauma Acute Care Surg 2014;76(4): 965–9.

24. Haydel MJ, Preston CA, Mills TJ, et al. Indications for computed tomography in patients with minor head injury. N Engl J Med 2000;343(2):100–5.

25. Cheng AL, Batool S, McCreary CR, et al. Susceptibility-weighted imaging is more reliable than T2*-weighted gradient-recalled echo MRI for detecting microbleeds. Stroke 2013;44(10):2782–6.

26. Goos JD, van der Flier WM, Knol DL, et al. Clinical relevance of improved microbleed detection by susceptibility-weighted magnetic resonance imaging. Stroke 2011;42(7):1894–900.

27. Shams S, Martola J, Cavallin L, et al. SWI or T2*: which MRI sequence to use in the detection of cerebral microbleeds? The Karolinska Imaging Dementia Study. AJNR Am J Neuroradiol 2015;36(6): 1089–95.

28. Beauchamp MH, Ditchfield M, Babl FE, et al. Detecting traumatic brain lesions in children: CT versus MRI versus susceptibility weighted imaging (SWI). J Neurotrauma 2011;28(6):915–27.

29. Tao JJ, Zhang WJ, Wang D, et al. Susceptibility weighted imaging in the evaluation of hemorrhagic diffuse axonal injury. Neural Regen Res 2015; 10(11):1879–81.

30. Trifan G, Gattu R, Haacke EM, et al. MR imaging findings in mild traumatic brain injury with persistent neurological impairment. Magn Reson Imaging 2017;37:243–51.

31. Maugans TA, Farley C, Altaye M, et al. Pediatric sports-related concussion produces cerebral blood flow alterations. Pediatrics 2012;129(1):28–37.

32. Jarrett M, Tam R, Hernandez-Torres E, et al. A prospective pilot investigation of brain volume, white matter hyperintensities, and hemorrhagic lesions after mild traumatic brain injury. Front Neurol 2016;7:11.

33. Hasiloglu ZI, Albayram S, Selcuk H, et al. Cerebral microhemorrhages detected by susceptibility-weighted imaging in amateur boxers. AJNR Am J Neuroradiol 2011;32(1):99–102.

34. Ellis MJ, Leiter J, Hall T, et al. Neuroimaging findings in pediatric sports-related concussion. J Neurosurg Pediatr 2015;16(3):241–7.

35. Yang Z, Yeo RA, Pena A, et al. An FMRI study of auditory orienting and inhibition of return in pediatric mild traumatic brain injury. J Neurotrauma 2012; 29(12):2124–36.

36. Sigmund GA, Tong KA, Nickerson JP, et al. Multimodality comparison of neuroimaging in pediatric traumatic brain injury. Pediatr Neurol 2007;36(4): 217–26.

37. Denk C, Rauscher A. Susceptibility weighted imaging with multiple echoes. J Magn Reson Imaging 2010;31(1):185–91.

38. Huang YL, Kuo YS, Tseng YC, et al. Susceptibility-weighted MRI in mild traumatic brain injury. Neurology 2015;84(6):580–5.

39. Wang X, Wei XE, Li MH, et al. Microbleeds on susceptibility-weighted MRI in depressive and non-depressive patients after mild traumatic brain injury. Neurol Sci 2014;35(10):1533–9.

40. Casson IR, Viano DC, Haacke EM, et al. Is there chronic brain damage in retired NFL players? Neuroradiology, neuropsychology, and neurology examinations of 45 retired players. Sports Health 2014;6(5):384–95.

41. Helmer KG, Pasternak O, Fredman E, et al. Hockey Concussion Education Project, part 1. Susceptibility-weighted imaging study in male and female ice hockey players over a single season. J Neurosurg 2014; 120(4):864–72.

42. Haacke EM, Tang J, Neelavalli J, et al. Susceptibility mapping as a means to visualize veins and quantify oxygen saturation. J Magn Reson Imaging 2010;32(3):663–76.

43. Chang K, Barnes S, Haacke EM, et al. Imaging the effects of oxygen saturation changes in voluntary apnea and hyperventilation on susceptibility-weighted imaging. AJNR Am J Neuroradiol 2014; 35(6):1091–5.

44. Tong KA, Ashwal S, Holshouser BA, et al. Diffuse axonal injury in children: clinical correlation with hemorrhagic lesions. Ann Neurol 2004;56(1): 36–50.

45. Chastain CA, Oyoyo UE, Zipperman M, et al. Predicting outcomes of traumatic brain injury by imaging modality and injury distribution. J Neurotrauma 2009;26(8):1183–96.

46. Barker P, Bizzi A, De Stefano N, et al. Pulse sequences and protocol design. Clinical MR spectroscopy, techniques and applications. Cambridge (United Kingdom): Cambridge University Press; 2010.

47. Mountford CE, Stanwell P, Lin A, et al. Neurospectroscopy: the past, present and future. Chem Rev 2010;110(5):3060–86.

48. Jansen JF, Backes WH, Nicolay K, et al. 1H MR spectroscopy of the brain: absolute quantification of metabolites. Radiology 2006;240(2):318–32.

49. Hoch SE, Kirov II, Tal A. When are metabolic ratios superior to absolute quantification? A statistical analysis. NMR Biomed 2017;30.

50. Simmons ML, Frondoza CG, Coyle JT. Immunocytochemical localization of N-acetyl-aspartate with monoclonal antibodies. Neuroscience 1991;45(1):37–45.

51. Baslow MH. N-acetylaspartate in the vertebrate brain: metabolism and function. Neurochem Res 2003;28(6):941–53.

52. Moffett JR, Ross B, Arun P, et al. N-Acetylaspartate in the CNS: from neurodiagnostics to neurobiology. Prog Neurobiol 2007;81(2):89–131.

53. Gujar S, Maheshwari S, Bjorkman-Burtscher I, et al. Magnetic resonance spectroscopy. J Neuroophthalmol 2005;25(3):217–26.

54. Govindaraju V, Gauger GE, Manley GT, et al. Volumetric proton spectroscopic imaging of mild traumatic brain injury. AJNR Am J Neuroradiol 2004; 25(5):730–7.

55. Lin AP, Liao HJ, Merugumala SK, et al. Metabolic imaging of mild traumatic brain injury. Brain Imaging Behav 2012;6(2):208–23.

56. Gasparovic C, Yeo R, Mannell M, et al. Neurometabolite concentrations in gray and white matter in mild traumatic brain injury: a 1HMagnetic resonance spectroscopy study. J Neurotrauma 2009; 26(10):1635–43.

57. Brand A, Richter-Landsberg C, Leibfritz D. Multinuclear NMR studies on the energy metabolism of glial and neuronal cells. Dev Neurosci 1993; 15(3–5):289–98.

58. Bitsch A, Bruhn H, Vougioukas V, et al. Inflammatory CNS demyelination: histopathologic correlation with in vivo quantitative proton MR spectroscopy. AJNR Am J Neuroradiol 1999; 20(9):1619–27.

59. De Graaf RA. In vivo NMR spectroscopy: principles and techniques. Chichester (UK): John Wiley & Sons Ltd; 2007. p. 61–2.

60. Prost RW, Mark L, Mewissen M, et al. Detection of glutamate/glutamine resonances by 1H magnetic resonance spectroscopy at 0.5 tesla. Magn Reson Med 1997;37(4):615–8.

61. Cecil KM, Hills EC, Sandel ME, et al. Proton magnetic resonance spectroscopy for detection of axonal injury in the splenium of the corpus callosum of brain-injured patients. J Neurosurg 1998;88(5):795–801.

62. Lin AP, Ramadan S, Stern RA, et al. Changes in the neurochemistry of athletes with repetitive brain trauma: preliminary results using localized correlated spectroscopy. Alzheimers Res Ther 2015; 7(1):13.

63. Narayana PA, Yu X, Hasan KM, et al. Multi-modal MRI of mild traumatic brain injury. Neuroimage Clin 2014;7:87–97.

64. Sours C, George EO, Zhuo J, et al. Hyper-connectivity of the thalamus during early stages following mild traumatic brain injury. Brain Imaging Behav 2015;9(3):550–63.

65. Henry LC, Tremblay S, Boulanger Y, et al. Neurometabolic changes in the acute phase after sports concussions correlate with symptom severity. J Neurotrauma 2010;27(1):65–76.

66. Poole VN, Abbas K, Shenk TE, et al. MR spectroscopic evidence of brain injury in the non-diagnosed collision sport athlete. Dev Neuropsychol 2014;39(6):459–73.

67. Dean PJ, Sato JR, Vieira G, et al. Multimodal imaging of mild traumatic brain injury and persistent postconcussion syndrome. Brain Behav 2015; 5(1):45–61.

68. Kierans AS, Kirov II, Gonen O, et al. Myoinositol and glutamate complex neurometabolite abnormality after mild traumatic brain injury. Neurology 2014;82(6):521–8.

69. George EO, Roys SR, Sours C, et al. Longitudinal and prognostic evaluation of mild traumatic brain injury: a 1H-MRS study. J Neurotrauma 2014; 31(11):1018–28.

70. Dhandapani S, Sharma A, Sharma K, et al. Comparative evaluation of MRS and SPECT in prognostication of patients with mild to moderate head injury. J Clin Neurosci 2014;21(5):745–50.

71. Vagnozzi R, Signoretti S, Cristofori L, et al. Assessment of metabolic brain damage and recovery following mild traumatic brain injury: a multicentre, proton magnetic resonance spectroscopic study in concussed patients. Brain 2010; 133(11):3232–42.

72. Sivak S, Bittsansky M, Grossmann J, et al. Clinical correlations of proton magnetic resonance spectroscopy findings in acute phase after mild traumatic brain injury. Brain Inj 2014;28(3):341–6.

73. Vagnozzi R, Signoretti S, Tavazzi B, et al. Temporal window of metabolic brain vulnerability to concussion: a pilot 1H-magnetic resonance spectroscopic study in concussed athletes–part III. Neurosurgery 2008;62(6):1286–95 [discussion: 95–6].

74. Yeo RA, Gasparovic C, Merideth F, et al. A longitudinal proton magnetic resonance spectroscopy study of mild traumatic brain injury. J Neurotrauma 2011;28(1):1–11.

75. Sarmento E, Moreira P, Brito C, et al. Proton spectroscopy in patients with post-traumatic headache attributed to mild head injury. Headache 2009; 49(9):1345–52.

76. Mayer AR, Ling JM, Dodd AB, et al. A longitudinal assessment of structural and chemical alterations in mixed martial arts fighters. J Neurotrauma 2015;32(22):1759–67.

77. Johnson B, Gay M, Zhang K, et al. The use of magnetic resonance spectroscopy in the subacute evaluation of athletes recovering from single and multiple mild traumatic brain injury. J Neurotrauma 2012;29(13):2297–304.

78. Johnson B, Zhang K, Gay M, et al. Metabolic alterations in corpus callosum may compromise brain functional connectivity in MTBI patients: an 1H-MRS study. Neurosci Lett 2012;509(1):5–8.

79. Cohen BA, Inglese M, Rusinek H, et al. Proton MR spectroscopy and MRI-volumetry in mild traumatic brain injury. AJNR Am J Neuroradiol 2007;28(5): 907–13.

80. Kirov II, Tal A, Babb JS, et al. Diffuse axonal injury in mild traumatic brain injury: a 3D multivoxel proton MR spectroscopy study. J Neurol 2013; 260(1):242–52.

81. Hetherington HP, Hamid H, Kulas J, et al. MRSI of the medial temporal lobe at 7 T in explosive blast mild traumatic brain injury. Magn Reson Med 2014;71(4):1358–67.

82. Maudsley AA, Govind V, Levin B, et al. Distributions of magnetic resonance diffusion and spectroscopy measures with traumatic brain injury. J Neurotrauma 2015;32(14):1056–63.

83. Koerte IK, Lin AP, Muehlmann M, et al. Altered neurochemistry in former professional soccer players without a history of concussion. J Neurotrauma 2015;32(17):1287–93.

84. Garnett MR, Blamire AM, Rajagopalan B, et al. Evidence for cellular damage in normal-appearing white matter correlates with injury severity in patients following traumatic brain injury: a magnetic resonance spectroscopy study. Brain 2000;123(Pt 7):1403–9.

85. Govind V, Gold S, Kaliannan K, et al. Whole-brain proton MR spectroscopic imaging of mild-to-moderate traumatic brain injury and correlation with neuropsychological deficits. J Neurotrauma 2010;27(3):483–96.

86. Vagnozzi R, Signoretti S, Floris R, et al. Decrease in N-acetylaspartate following concussion may be coupled to decrease in creatine. J Head Trauma Rehabil 2013;28(4):284–92.

87. Ashwal S, Holshouser B, Tong K, et al. Proton spectroscopy detected myoinositol in children with traumatic brain injury. Pediatr Res 2004;56(4):630–8.

88. Shutter L, Tong KA, Holshouser BA. Proton MRS in acute traumatic brain injury: role for glutamate/ glutamine and choline for outcome prediction. J Neurotrauma 2004;21(12):1693–705.

89. Chamard E, Lassonde M, Henry L, et al. Neurometabolic and microstructural alterations following a sports-related concussion in female athletes. Brain Inj 2013;27(9):1038–46.

90. Kirov I, Fleysher L, Babb JS, et al. Characterizing 'mild' in traumatic brain injury with proton MR spectroscopy in the thalamus: initial findings. Brain Inj 2007;21(11):1147–54.

91. Tremblay S, Beaule V, Proulx S, et al. Multimodal assessment of primary motor cortex integrity following sport concussion in asymptomatic athletes. Clin Neurophysiol 2014; 125(7):1371–9.

92. Henry LC, Tremblay S, Leclerc S, et al. Metabolic changes in concussed American football players during the acute and chronic post-injury phases. BMC Neurol 2011;11:105.

93. Lipton ML, Kim N, Zimmerman ME, et al. Soccer heading is associated with white matter microstructural and cognitive abnormalities. Radiology 2013; 268(3):850–7.

94. Garnett MR, Blamire AM, Corkill RG, et al. Early proton magnetic resonance spectroscopy in normal-appearing brain correlates with outcome in patients following traumatic brain injury. Brain 2000;123(Pt 10):2046–54.

95. Sinson G, Bagley LJ, Cecil KM, et al. Magnetization transfer imaging and proton MR spectroscopy in the evaluation of axonal injury: correlation with clinical outcome after traumatic brain injury. AJNR Am J Neuroradiol 2001;22(1):143–51.

96. Uzan M, Albayram S, Dashti SG, et al. Thalamic proton magnetic resonance spectroscopy in vegetative state induced by traumatic brain injury. J Neurol Neurosurg Psychiatry 2003; 74(1):33–8.

97. Holshouser BA, Tong KA, Ashwal S, et al. Prospective longitudinal proton magnetic resonance spectroscopic imaging in adult traumatic brain injury. J Magn Reson Imaging 2006;24(1):33–40.

98. Tollard E, Galanaud D, Perlbarg V, et al. Experience of diffusion tensor imaging and 1H spectroscopy for outcome prediction in severe traumatic brain injury: preliminary results. Crit Care Med 2009; 37(4):1448–55.

99. Aaen GS, Holshouser BA, Sheridan C, et al. Magnetic resonance spectroscopy predicts outcomes for children with nonaccidental trauma. Pediatrics 2010;125(2):295–303.

100. Holshouser BA, Tong KA, Ashwal S. Proton MR spectroscopic imaging depicts diffuse axonal injury in children with traumatic brain injury. AJNR Am J Neuroradiol 2005;26(5):1276–85.

101. Danielsen ER, Christensen PB, Arlien-Soborg P, et al. Axonal recovery after severe traumatic brain

injury demonstrated in vivo by 1H MR spectroscopy. Neuroradiology 2003;45(10):722–4.

102. Belli A, Sen J, Petzold A, et al. Extracellular *N*-acetylaspartate depletion in traumatic brain injury. J Neurochem 2006;96(3):861–9.

103. Signoretti S, Marmarou A, Tavazzi B, et al. *N*-Acetylaspartate reduction as a measure of injury severity and mitochondrial dysfunction following diffuse traumatic brain injury. J Neurotrauma 2001;18(10): 977–91.

104. Kirov II, Tal A, Babb JS, et al. Proton MR spectroscopy correlates diffuse axonal abnormalities with post-concussive symptoms in mild traumatic brain injury. J Neurotrauma 2013;30(13):1200–4.

105. Widerstrom-Noga E, Govind V, Adcock JP, et al. Subacute pain after traumatic brain injury is associated with lower insular *N*-acetylaspartate concentrations. J Neurotrauma 2016;33(14):1380–9.

106. Friedman SD, Brooks WM, Jung RE, et al. Quantitative proton MRS predicts outcome after traumatic brain injury. Neurology 1999;52(7):1384–91.

107. Benarroch EE. *N*-acetylaspartate and *N*-acetylaspartylglutamate: neurobiology and clinical significance. Neurology 2008;70(16):1353–7.

108. Signoretti S, Lazzarino G, Tavazzi B, et al. The pathophysiology of concussion. PM R 2011;3(10 Suppl 2):S359–68.

109. Vagnozzi R, Tavazzi B, Signoretti S, et al. Temporal window of metabolic brain vulnerability to concussions: mitochondrial-related impairment–part I. Neurosurgery 2007;61(2):379–88 [discussion: 88–9].

Functional MR Imaging: Blood Oxygen Level–Dependent and Resting State Techniques in Mild Traumatic Brain Injury

Scott Rosenthal, MS[a,b], Matthew Gray, BS[a,b],
Hudaisa Fatima, MSc[a,b], Haris I. Sair, MD, PhD[c],
Christopher T. Whitlow, MD, PhD, MHA[a,b,d,e,*]

KEYWORDS

- Functional MR imaging • Blood oxygen level dependent • Resting state • Mild traumatic brain injury

KEY POINTS

- There are numerous changes in resting state functional MR imaging postconcussion.
- Although the overall time-course of mTBI-associated effects on functional connectivity are still being elucidated, some general trends with respect to initial injury, persistent change and recovery have begun to emerge in the literature.
- There seems to be a period of acute post-injury default mode network hyperconnectivity, followed by a period of decreased connectivity before later connectivity normalization in some patients.

INTRODUCTION

Concussions are clinically diagnosed from behavioral observations, patient-reported symptoms, and physical examination. Neurocognitive testing may be used and is often helpful; however, it is not required for diagnosis. No biomarkers to reliably diagnose concussion have been incorporated into routine clinical practice, and conventional neuroimaging methods are typically negative.

Furthermore, the same limitations that exist for initial diagnosis are also present in monitoring recovery.[1] Functional MR (fMR) imaging is an evolving form of neuroimaging that permits quantitative measurement of brain function that may one day aid diagnosis and can be repeated longitudinally for evaluation of recovery.[2] It has been posited that fMR imaging is a more sensitive tool for postconcussion neuropsychological evaluation than classic testing methods.[3]

[a] Radiology Informatics and Image Processing Laboratory (RIIPL), Wake Forest School of Medicine, Medical Center Boulevard, Winston-Salem, NC 27157, USA; [b] Division of Neuroradiology, Department of Radiology, Wake Forest School of Medicine, Medical Center Boulevard, Winston-Salem, NC 27157, USA; [c] Division of Neuroradiology, The Russell H. Morgan Department of Radiology and Radiological Sciences, Johns Hopkins University School of Medicine, 601 North Caroline Street, Baltimore, MD 21205, USA; [d] Department of Biomedical Engineering, Wake Forest School of Medicine, Medical Center Boulevard, Winston-Salem, NC 27157, USA; [e] Clinical Translational Sciences Institute (CTSI), Wake Forest School of Medicine, Medical Center Boulevard, Winston-Salem, NC 27157, USA
* Corresponding author. Department of Radiology, Department of Biomedical Engineering, Clinical Translational Sciences Institute, Wake Forest School of Medicine, Medical Center Boulevard, Winston-Salem, NC 27157-1088.
E-mail address: cwhitlow@wakehealth.edu

Neuroimag Clin N Am 28 (2018) 107–115
https://doi.org/10.1016/j.nic.2017.09.008
1052-5149/18/© 2017 Elsevier Inc. All rights reserved.

fMR imaging quantifies brain activity based on the relationship between neural activity and localized hemodynamic responses. Although the exact mechanism has not been determined, neural activity typically induces a hemodynamic response that results in a net effect of increased oxyhemoglobin level in relation to deoxyhemoglobin level in the local microvasculature. With increased ratio of oxyhemoglobin to deoxyhemoglobin, there is a reduction in local magnetic susceptibility, which can be measured using blood oxygen level–dependent (BOLD) contrast where increased signal results.

There are 2 broad approaches to using this BOLD contrast in functional neuroimaging. In task-fMR imaging, a specific sensorimotor or cognitive task is performed by the patient, and correlations of BOLD signal with task modulation are computed. Any brain region that shows BOLD oscillations that are synchronous with the performance of the task are considered to be relevant to performance of that task. More recently, a task-free paradigm has emerged, now described as resting state fMR (rs-fMR) imaging, in which the patient does not perform a specific task while BOLD images are acquired. The patient thus engages in undirected processes throughout the acquisition. Despite this lack of task-oriented cognitive control through the acquisition, fairly consistent spatial patterns of temporal BOLD correlations have been shown using rs-fMR imaging. Spatially distinct regions of the brain that show temporally synchronous BOLD signal (and by inference neural activity) have been characterized as various intrinsic resting state brain networks.[4]

There are significant benefits of rs-fMR imaging compared with task-fMR imaging. Because no task is explicitly performed in rs-fMR imaging, this technique can be used to negate the confounding issue of patient performance, which can be variable depending on the population that is being studied. This advantage lends itself to greater uniformity in data acquisition if the imaging parameters are kept constant across sites. Furthermore, with task-fMR imaging, only a specific subset of cognitive processes are interrogated; in contrast, rs-fMR imaging provides information about multiple brain networks across the entire brain. Given the ease of acquisition compared with task-fMR imaging, as well as the breadth of information acquired, rs-fMR imaging has in most cases supplanted task-fMR imaging for investigation of brain function across a wide variety of brain disorders; and this article therefore focuses on rs-fMR imaging in the context of concussions.

Alterations of functional connectivity assessed by rs-fMR imaging are described with respect to the chronology of presentation, starting with the immediate postconcussive time frame and extending to years postinjury. In addition, this article uses the terms mild traumatic brain injury (mTBI) and concussion interchangeably, although there is active debate about the specific meaning of these terms in both the clinical and research domains.

ACUTE MILD TRAUMATIC BRAIN INJURY

In the recent literature, the acute phase of an mTBI is typically considered the initial 30-day period postinjury. The time period immediately following an mTBI is characterized by rapid changes in which the brain presumably attempts to recover from the initial concussive insult. rs-fMR imaging has shown variable patterns depending on the timing of imaging in the acute phase.[5] This variability is understandable because both the primary injury and early inflammatory response occur during this period and subsequently begin to heal.[6] The primary injury is a direct result of impact exposure and may include primarily axonal injury resulting from the sudden deformation of brain. The inflammatory response follows this neuronal injury as edema, neurotransmitter release, and vascular dysfunction. This early time period can be particularly difficult for patients as they attempt to manage their symptoms, which often include headache, cognitive fogging, emotional lability, insomnia, and slowed reaction times.[7] Although almost all concussive symptoms resolve within 10 days, some patients can be burdened with a more prolonged postconcussive syndrome (PCS) that can continue for months and even years. For young athletes busy in both athletics and academics, the immediate postconcussive period can be particularly stressful because their return to play depends on a successful return to school.

In the setting of all this neurocognitive change, rs-fMR imaging attempts to provide imaging correlates of concussion and relate them to concussive symptoms, time postinjury, degree of recovery, and other variables in order to characterize the brain-related functional impact of injury. Through repeated imaging across the acute and chronic phases of injury, some trends have begun to emerge, showing an expected pattern of mTBI recovery compared with large control groups. Most consistently explored are the default mode network (DMN) and task-positive networks (TPNs). The DMN primarily consists of coordinated activities of the posterior cingulate cortex, medial prefrontal cortex, hippocampus, and parahippocampus, and it has been described to be involved in introspection, memory, planning, and daydreaming.[8] In contrast, the TPN is anticorrelated with the DMN and is typically active during external, goal-driven tasks.[9] Patients with mTBI have been reported to have worse than average headaches, suggesting an association between post-mTBI headache and DMN connectivity.[10]

In the first 3 to 5 days following an mTBI, fMR imaging studies have shown increased functional connectivity and cerebral blood flow (CBF) of key DMN regions, such as the hippocampus. This direction of change is in contrast with the decreased functional connectivity within these regions, which is often seen on fMR imaging at later stages.[5,10,11] The reason for this is not yet known; however, variability in the mechanism by which the impact is transmitted to the head may explain some of this inconsistency as well as the wide range of post-concussive symptoms that often arise.

Although it is possible that the increases in CBF and connectivity may reflect a short-term compensatory mechanism during the first few days postinjury, it has also been postulated that the shock from trauma alters cerebrovascular reactivity within the brain.[10] This altered cerebrovascular control may then affect fMR imaging measures of functional connectivity yielding changes that are unrelated to neuronal function, and possibly representing a mismatch in metabolic demand and supply during this phase. Alternatively, it is possible that decreased synchronization of neurons results in a need for heightened connectivity in order to create the same signal.[12] This higher connectivity is likely to require greater CBF to meet the increased metabolic requirements. In addition, it is important to remember that the secondary effects of injury may also occur during this period, with altered blood flow and connectivity patterns that begin to manifest as subsequent recovery begins. It is also possible that the effects of prior concussions could modulate patterns of connectivity associated with acute traumatic brain injury, although one recent study reported that there was no fMR imaging evidence that prior concussions altered observed connectivity patterns.[5] However, this presumption needs additional investigation, because many studies exclude participants with previous concussions to avoid confounding.

Some studies have examined regional homogeneity (ReHo) in addition to global brain connectivity (GBC) via fMR imaging during the first week post-mTBI. ReHo is a measure of the connectivity of immediately neighboring voxels, compared with functional connectivity estimates that have no spatial constraints.[12] Although no mTBI-related changes were found in GBC, significantly reduced ReHo was seen in the left insula, which is an important relay for cognitive switching from resting state to TPNs. This pattern of connectivity correlated with the Mini-Mental State Examination scores, which suggests that these functional brain findings are associated with cognitive sequelae.[13]

Following the initial period of injury, fMR imaging connectivity continues to change, even as the initial associated symptoms begin to resolve. By approximately weeks 1 to 2 postinjury, most patients are asymptomatic and often feel as though they have returned to their baselines. Although these patients have been shown to be cognitively normal by neurocognitive testing and clinically asymptomatic, many show deficits on both task-oriented fMR imaging and rs-fMR imaging.[14]

Beginning around week 1 post-mTBI, the initial increased connectivity of the DMN observed during the first few days after injury decreases, with diminished interhemispheric functional connectivity (IH-FC).[15,16] In addition, functional connections within the DMN and communication with the TPN have been shown to be significantly reduced or absent.[17] These decreases are generally seen in both patients who are asymptomatic clinically and those still reporting dysfunction.[16] Importantly, reductions in IH-FC were predicted by impaired performance on neurocognitive testing. There seems to be a dose-dependent effect of prior concussions on functional connectivity of the DMN, because patients showed decreased number and strength of DMN connections in relation to their prior number of concussions.[17] Some additional studies have suggested decreased interhemispheric connectivity of the hippocampus and parahippocampus in the setting of decreased whole-brain connectivity; however, others have been unable to replicate such findings. Little consensus exists as to what additional network changes occur within this time period, and, even within the well-characterized DMN, controversy still exists.[15,18,19]

Several studies have attempted to unmask hidden deficits by observing the resting brain following the YMCA stress test. Between weeks 1 and 2, when patients were asymptomatic based on clinical and neuropsychiatric testing, significant decreases in DMN functional connectivity were shown following physical exertion despite non–significantly different baseline scans.[20,21] These results suggest that previously undetectable dysfunction can be revealed with physical stress; however, the clinical significance of this dysfunction remains to be determined.

Looking beyond resting state networks, some information can be gleaned from TPNs. Clearly, the impact of mTBI extends beyond the DMN to other networks and areas of the brain, which may become dysfunctional during the same event or alter their function to compensate in some manner to maintain function.[16] In one study, patients with persistent cognitive symptoms 1 week postinjury required greater activation of the TPN to achieve similar performance on simple tasks.[22] Asymptomatic patients also seemed to have greater activation of regions outside the DMN, possibly representing compensatory recruitment.[22,23]

Longitudinal studies have suggested that compensation and healing begin as early as day 10 postconcussion. These studies have been important in correlating imaging findings with PCS symptoms and neurocognitive testing. In one recent study, rs-fMR imaging of patients acquired 1 to 2 weeks post-mTBI correlated with cognitive performance and risk of developing of PCS.[19,23] The magnitude of decrease in DMN functional connectivity correlated with persistent symptoms. PCS represents persistent concussive-induced symptoms including, but not limited to, permanent mental fog, irritability, cognitive difficulties, headaches, and/or even the development of depression. The risk of PCS after mTBI ranges from 10% in young individuals to more than 50% in older individuals.[24] Because is it is speculated that recovery from mTBI is mediated by compensatory connectivity, it is possible that the brain loses this ability with age.[19]

Longitudinal fMR imaging studies in particular have begun to characterize how the brain recovers following mTBI, including increased connectivity in the immediate postconcussive phase (days 1–5), subsequent decrease in connectivity during the subacute phase (days 7–14), and then normalization as the subacute stage begins (day 30). It is possible that, one day, rs-fMR imaging performed in the window of 1 to 2 weeks may be able to predict (1) recovery from mTBI, and (2) development of PCS depending on the magnitude or pattern of network connectivity change.

SUBACUTE MILD TRAUMATIC BRAIN INJURY

In the subacute phase, several recent studies have incorporated rs-fMR imaging and task-based fMR imaging paradigms to delineate functional connectivity and activation changes post-mTBI. In the time frame marking the initial stages of this phase, within 21 to 32 days postinjury, prominent alterations in functional properties have been noted.

Network Connectivity Assessments

Small-worldness is a graph theoretic analysis measure that refers to a pattern of connectivity in which neighboring nodes are directly connected and distant nodes are also connected, which is thought to allow increased efficiency in interneuronal communication.[25] Graph theoretic

analyses measuring small-worldness have shown a decrease in exchange of information at the global level and an increase in communication among neighboring nodes. This finding has been proposed to reflect increased local efficiency among local neurons and decreased global efficiency of distant connections.[26] A secondary analysis by these investigators using diffusion tensor imaging found these whole-brain differences to be related to diffuse axonal injury. Reduced anisotropy was noted reflecting possible damage to white matter fibers in frontal and occipital regions. Moreover, anatomic and whole-brain correlations between global efficiency and regional anisotropy suggested a distributed pattern of functional network dysfunction. The investigators suggested a mechanism of structural damage preceding this connectivity disruption. Identification of the potential mechanisms underlying network level dysfunction still warrants further examination. Emerging research also denotes dysregulation of CBF as a contributory process to concussion pathophysiology.[27] Inadequate CBF resulting in a failure to match the metabolic demands of the brain have been shown to affect mTBI outcomes through a process of secondary brain injury.[28] Hence, inclusion of sensitive CBF measures in future analyses is needed to understand injury mechanisms and predict outcomes.

Xiong and colleagues[29] found alterations in spontaneous neural activity in patients by evaluating amplitudes of low-frequency fluctuations (ALFFs). ALFFs reflect the intensity of spontaneous neuronal activity in a brain region, and mTBI-associated changes of this activity have been proposed to reflect brain dysfunction.[29] A significant relationship between ALFF of the cingulate gyrus and a measure of working memory was shown in patients with mTBI. This finding suggests that decreased ALFFs may result in poorer working memory post-mTBI. Decreased hippocampal connectivity was also significantly associated with poorer working memory performance. In addition, decreased functional connectivity pairs were found in the thalamus, left caudate nucleus, and right hippocampus.

At 2 months postinjury, Stevens and colleagues[30] conducted functional connectivity assessments of 15 resting state networks using independent component analysis. Altered patterns of connectivity strength were found among all networks tested. Abnormal connectivity was noted between frontoparietal, frontotemporal, and interhemispheric sites. Diminished connectivity in anterior cingulate cortex (ACC) was also found to be mediated by number of PCS complaints. ACC has a variety of functional roles, including pain processing, cognitive control, conflict monitoring, and emotional processing.[31] As such, diminished connectivity involving ACC may serve as an underlying neural mechanism contributing toward the development of PCS.

Thalamocortical Connections

Literature examining thalamocortical connectivity associated with subacute mTBI reports inconsistencies in the direction of connectivity. For instance, Zhou and colleagues[26] found higher thalamocortical connectivity in patients with mTBI during the subacute phase postinjury, but a previous study by the same authors describes contradictory findings.[32] In the 2014 study, Zhou and colleagues[32] used fractional low-frequency fluctuations (fALFF) instead of conventional functional connectivity MR (fcMR) imaging to assess thalamocortical connections that are time delayed. Reduced fALFF in the thalamus was found, along with subregions projecting to frontal and temporal cortices. Lower connectivity between thalamofrontal and thalamotemporal regions were also found. Patients also showed reduced connectivity between the thalamus and motor/supplementary motor regions in response to a finger-tapping task, compared with controls. Xiong and colleagues[29] also showed this reduced thalamic connectivity, but with the left middle frontal gyrus (MFG). Disparities in these results may be explained by use of different image preprocessing steps and fcMR imaging data analysis.

At 1.5 months post-mTBI, Banks and colleagues[33] investigated functional connectivity between the thalamus and 3 of the brain's resting state networks: (1) the DMN, (2) the anticorrelated dorsal attentional network (DAN), and (3) the frontoparietal control network (FPC). Patients showed increased functional connectivity between thalamus-DMN; however, connectivity between thalamus-DAN and thalamus-FPC was decreased. Patients also experienced higher pain intensity and posttraumatic stress disorder (PTSD) symptoms compared with controls. Changes after a 4-month follow-up provided insights into clinical recovery, with normalization of thalamus-DAN connectivity; however, thalamus-DMN connections further increased away from patients' baselines, which may have been related to PTSD symptoms. Similar evidence supporting this hypothesis was reported in patients with earthquake-related trauma from a cohort of survivors who developed symptoms of PTSD and showed increased thalamus-DMN connectivity 8 months post-TBI.

Default Mode Network Connectivity After Mild Traumatic Brain Injury

Diminished connectivity has been reported in regions generally encompassing the DMN.[30] This decreased connectivity correlated positively with PCS complaints. However, one specific region of the DMN, the precuneus, showed increased connectivity in this analysis, and this increase was inversely related to the extent of PCS complaints. Among the scarcity of longitudinal studies in the mTBI literature, Bharath and colleagues[34] reported time-dependent changes in resting state functional connectivity between patients without PCS complaints compared with controls. Most connectivity changes were found to occur between 3 and 6 months postinjury. Patients showed decreased DMN connectivity at 3 months, as opposed to 36 hours postinjury when DMN hyperconnectivity was observed. Nathan and colleagues[1] described abnormal patterns of hyperconnectivity within the DMN (ACC, left and right posterior cingulate cortex [PCC], and temporal regions) that were identified 5 months postinjury. The investigators also provided valuable insights into the various confounds that need to be examined within mTBI studies, and that likely contribute to the inconsistent functional injury outcomes reported across the current literature. Specifically, injury severity, location, and time since injury were found to alter DMN connectivity.

Speculations on Compensatory Mechanisms

Higher local efficiency within 21 to 32 days has been shown to be negatively correlated with PCS scores and lower global efficiency.[26] These associations have been interpreted to reflect a possible compensatory upregulation present to preserve postinjury functioning. Xiong and colleagues[29] also found significantly increased ALFF in parieto-occipital regions. Iraji and colleagues[35] described a compensatory response pattern within the DMN, showing hyperconnectivity of the PCC with frontal lobe and the supplementary motor area (SMA), which was associated with increased environmental awareness and PCS symptoms.[36] More research is necessary to determine whether this increase in connectivity represents additional compensatory brain region recruitment or hyperactivity associated with abnormal response patterns post-mTBI.

At 2 months after mTBI, Stevens and colleagues[30] found evidence for increased regional connectivity in various resting state networks. These networks included the secondary visual processing network, limbic circuit, and cingulo-opercular network. The precuneus also showed increased strength of integration within the DMN, as previously mentioned. In addition to increased regional connectivity, nonnetwork brain regions were reported to be recruited alongside the typical networks; for example, the frontoparietal regions (typically part of executive networks) were more integrated with the limbic network. Previous studies have described such patterns of connectivity as possibly reflecting the ability of the brain to adapt network responses for optimal functioning after injury.[37] More complementary evidence of functional recovery via regional network recruitment was reported by Bharath and colleagues.[34] Initial DMN hyperconnectivity spread to other brain areas after 3 months. After 6 months, patients without PCS were reported to have neuropsychological test scores that were comparable with controls. There is considerable need for future studies to include analyses between regions of hyperconnectivity and neuropsychological batteries in order to better classify the compensatory processes post-mTBI.

Czerniack and colleagues[2] showed functional compensation through increased connection strength between the ACC; a DMN node; and areas comprising the executive control network, salience network, as well as the left and right dorsolateral prefrontal cortex (DLPFC). There were no group differences between patients and controls on measures of executive function. Furthermore, better performance on measures of inhibition positively correlated with connectivity between the ACC and right middle frontal, left DLPFC, and right inferior parietal regions.

Neurocognitive Outcomes

Because of the heterogeneous nature of fMR imaging studies, with only a few using neuropsychological tests, the relationship between cognitive measures and changes in functional connectivity remains unclear. Higher thalamocortical activity correlated with increased local efficiency.[32] This finding was interpreted to indicate dysfunctional connectivity resulting in decreased efficiency in neuronal usage. Aberrant thalamocortical connectivity has previously been associated with memory dysfunction and behavioral complaints in epilepsy.[38] Incorporation of sensitive cognitive tests in future fMR imaging connectivity studies is necessary to elucidate the relationship between thalamocortical activity, neuronal usage, and cognitive dysfunction. Decreased network connectivity between the left thalamus and left MFG was positively correlated with measures of working memory in patients with mTBI.[29] Decreased ALFF in cingulate gyrus also positively correlated with these measures of working memory. These findings are interesting, because the cingulate

gyrus has been reported to regulate functions associated with emotion, learning, and memory.[29]

Positive correlations have been described between DMN hyperconnected regions and measures of depression, aggression, and stress-related symptoms. These alterations were thought to reflect limitations in the modulation of emotions and attention, resulting in increased efforts to relax even in the absence of demanding stimuli. Deficits were also found in verbal learning and memory, reaction time, sustained attention, and mental switching. The DMN is known to deactivate during active task performance. In addition, when time since injury was regressed out, DMN hyperconnectivity correlated with these neuropsychological measures.

CHRONIC MILD TRAUMATIC BRAIN INJURY

It has been postulated that most functional recovery occurs in the first 3 to 6 month postinjury and that normalization of fMR imaging may be representative of uncomplicated recovery postconcussion.[34] In this small study examining recovery, DMN hyperconnectivity was reported in the immediate days following injury.[34] These same subjects then proceeded to develop decreased DMN connectivity at 3 months that correlated with poorer neurocognitive performance. At 6 months, these subjects had functional connectivity that was not significantly different from that of healthy controls. As these subjects' fMR imaging connectivity normalized, so did their neurocognitive performance.[34] In contrast, continued PCS symptoms at 6 months and poorer performance on tasks involving attention, processing speed, and cognitive flexibility have been shown to correlate with decreased DMN connectivity.[23] These findings suggest that prolonged concussion recovery is related to a failure to normalize neural networks.

The absence of concussive symptoms and normalization of clinical neurocognitive performance does not guarantee complete concussion resolution. Patients examined 7.5 months postinjury showed no notable difference in neurocognitive performance compared with healthy controls, but fMR imaging analysis yielded significantly increased connectivity within the frontoparietal working memory circuit and recruitment of additional regions outside this network.[39] This increased connectivity and activation suggests increased cognitive effort in order to compensate for continued deficits in function. Such compensation sufficiently hides deficits, resulting in normal-appearing neurocognitive function.[39] This phenomenon, known as cognitive reserve, is characterized by recruitment of additional cognitive resources to compensate for neurologic dysfunction.[40] This phenomenon is also thought to play a role in the development of chronic traumatic encephalopathy, which is a neurodegenerative disorder thought to be related to head impact exposure.[41] Based on this theory, individuals never fully recovery from injury. Instead, they accumulate additional injuries that slowly diminish cognitive resources until deficits overwhelm cognitive reserve and become clinically apparent.[40] Research regarding the underlying pathophysiologic mechanism is still underway.

A study examining 15 asymptomatic subjects with a mean of approximately 40 months postconcussion found decreased functional connectivity within the anterior DMN, increased activity within the posterior DMN, and increased activity of areas outside the DMN. Again, this increased activation suggests a compensatory mechanism permitting the appearance of clinical recovery.[42] It has also been hypothesized that increased posterior DMN activity may be part of normal recovery, because other studies have found the opposite to be associated with persistent psychiatric complaints.[42] When inadequate functional network compensation exists, patients often report continued neuropsychological and neurocognitive complaints, which has been observed in the blast-induced mTBI literature. Although the mechanism of blast-induced mTBI differs greatly from that of standard civilian concussions, the overall premise may be comparable. Decreased connectivity in the frontal lobes, visual system, and DMN have been observed 1 to 5 years after blast-induced mTBI.[43] Decreased frontal and visual connectivity was significantly associated with poorer measures of executive function and increased severity of patients' PCS symptoms. Increasing severity of blast-induced mTBI was also significantly associated with decreased connectivity, suggesting a relationship between severity of injury and risk of PCS. The number of blast-induced mTBIs was also inversely related to the connectivity of the precuneus, which is a key node within the DMN.[43] Weaker DMN connectivity has been observed in an additional blast-induced mTBI study[44] in which the functional connectivity of the DMN correlated with poorer attention and processing speed. It was speculated that the decreased connectivity within the DMN results in a lag of activation or incomplete activation resulting in deficits and contributing to PCS complaints. These subjects also had higher bilateral temporoparietal activity and decreased activity of the left inferior temporal region compared with controls. The tempoparietal regions are involved in vigilance, and it has been suggested that hyperconnectivity in this region

may play a role in the development of PTSD following blast-induced mTBI.[44]

Clinically, PCS and PTSD have significant overlap and it has been proposed that these two syndromes exist along a spectrum of post-mTBI dysfunction.[44] One study sought to further categorize these syndromes 5 years after blast-induced mTBI by sorting subjects into 2 groups and then comparing them with healthy controls. This categorization resulted in the formation of 3 groups: (1) subjects with PCS and PTSD, (2) subjects with PCS, and (3) healthy controls. The PCS and PTSD group had significantly higher connectivity between the left striatum and right hippocampus compared with the PCS-only group, and the PCS-only group had significantly increased connectivity compared with the healthy controls. Increased connectivity also correlated with poorer neurocognitive functioning, suggesting that higher connectivity is associated with greater symptom burden. This finding somewhat supports the theory that PCS and PTSD exist as a spectrum because the PCS-only group had abnormal but reduced activation of the same region as the PCS and PTSD group. To further categorize this relationship, the study reorganized the 3 groups based on the strength of connectivity between the striatum and hippocampus. This reorganization resulted in some overlap at the edges of these groups, suggesting a more spectrumlike existence of dysfunction.[45]

In addition to the striatum and hippocampus, the thalamus has been implicated in PCS complaints.[44,46] A study examining subjects 5 years postinjury found decreased functional connectivity of the thalamus after a 20-minute vigilance task. This decreased connectivity was inversely related to subjects' self-reported level of cognitive fatigue. Reaction time was also significantly slowed after the vigilance task. The thalamus represents an information relay station of the brain and direct communication to numerous subcortical regions.[46] As such, dysfunction of the thalamus could result in the generalized cognitive complaint of fatigue and prolonged reaction time. Similar results have been shown in a study examining blast-induced mTBI up to 5 years postinjury. One study found thalamic dysfunction that was significantly associated with poorer neurocognitive performance.[43]

Although there is still much to learn about the long-term effects of concussion, it seems that the persistence of abnormal functional connectivity is related to continued neurocognitive and neuropsychiatric complaints. In addition, such deficits and complaint are present up to 5 years postinjury and likely persist longer.

SUMMARY

There are numerous changes in rs-fMR imaging postconcussion. Although the overall pattern of initial injury, recovery, and healing are still being elucidated, some general trends have emerged in the literature. There seems to be a period of hyper-connectivity of the DMN in the immediate days following a concussion. The weeks after this initial stage are followed by a period of decreased connectivity, and then some patients begin to show normalization of fMR imaging connectivity patterns. Those with network connectivity patterns that do not normalize have been reported to develop PCS, PTSD, and/or neuropsychiatric complaints that may be related to alterations in connectivity of key regions of the DMN. However, there is limited agreement on the direction of these network connectivity changes in the current literature. However, it seems that these abnormalities may remain evident up to 5 years postinjury and potentially longer.

Much variation exists in the current literature regarding the natural progression of connectivity postinjury. One possible explanation for this variation in reported network connectivity findings post-TBI is that they may reflect the heterogeneity of study design. Future studies should target imaging to distinct time points, standardize imaging protocols, increase sample sizes, and apply stringent exclusion criteria to reduce the numerous confounders that exist.

REFERENCES

1. Nathan DE, Oakes TR, Yeh PH, et al. Exploring variations in functional connectivity of the resting state default mode network in mild traumatic brain injury. Brain connectivity 2015;5(2):102–14.
2. Czerniak SM, Sikoglu EM, Liso Navarro AA, et al. A resting state functional magnetic resonance imaging study of concussion in collegiate athletes. Brain Imaging Behav 2015;9(2):323–32.
3. Toth A. Chapter 24. Magnetic resonance imaging application in the area of mild and acute traumatic brain injury: implications for diagnostic markers?. In: Kobeissy FH, editor. Brain neurotrauma: molecular, neuropsychological, and rehabilitation aspects. Boca Raton (FL): CRC Press/Taylor & Francis; 2015. p. 329–40.
4. Fox MD, Snyder AZ, Vincent JL, et al. The human brain is intrinsically organized into dynamic, anticorrelated functional networks. Proc Natl Acad Sci U S A 2005;102(27):9673–8.
5. Churchill NW, Hutchison MG, Richards D, et al. The first week after concussion: blood flow, brain function and white matter microstructure. Neuroimage Clin 2017;14:480–9.
6. da Costa L, van Niftrik CB, Crane D, et al. Temporal profile of cerebrovascular reactivity impairment, gray matter volumes, and persistent symptoms after mild traumatic head injury. Front Neurol 2016;7:70.
7. McCrory P, Meeuwisse WH, Aubry M, et al. Consensus statement on concussion in sport: the 4th International Conference on Concussion in Sport held in Zurich, November 2012. Br J Sports Med 2013;47(5):250–8.
8. Zhu DC, Majumdar S. Integration of resting-state FMRI and diffusion-weighted MRI connectivity analyses of the human brain: limitations and improvement. J Neuroimaging 2014;24(2):176–86.
9. Sours C, Zhuo J, Janowich J, et al. Default mode network interference in mild traumatic brain injury - a pilot resting state study. Brain Res 2013;1537:201–15.
10. Militana AR, Donahue MJ, Sills AK, et al. Alterations in default-mode network connectivity may be influenced by cerebrovascular changes within 1 week of sports related concussion in college varsity athletes: a pilot study. Brain Imaging Behav 2016; 10(2):559–68.
11. Zhu DC, Covassin T, Nogle S, et al. A potential biomarker in sports-related concussion: brain functional connectivity alteration of the default-mode network measured with longitudinal resting-state fMRI over thirty days. J Neurotrauma 2015;32(5):327–41.
12. Meier TB, Bellgowan PS, Mayer AR. Longitudinal assessment of local and global functional connectivity following sports-related concussion. Brain Imaging Behav 2016;11(1):129–40.
13. Zhan J, Gao L, Zhou F, et al. Decreased regional homogeneity in patients with acute mild traumatic brain injury: a resting-state fMRI study. J Nervous Ment Dis 2015;203(10):786–91.
14. Lovell MR, Pardini JE, Welling J, et al. Functional brain abnormalities are related to clinical recovery and time to return-to-play in athletes. Neurosurgery 2007;61(2):352–9.
15. Iraji A, Benson RR, Welch RD, et al. Resting state functional connectivity in mild traumatic brain injury at the acute stage: independent component and seed-based analyses. J Neurotrauma 2015;32(14):1031–45.
16. Sours C, Chen H, Roys S, et al. Investigation of multiple frequency ranges using discrete wavelet decomposition of resting-state functional connectivity in mild traumatic brain injury patients. Brain Connectivity 2015;5(7):442–50.
17. Johnson B, Zhang K, Gay M, et al. Alteration of brain default network in subacute phase of injury in concussed individuals: resting-state fMRI study. Neuroimage 2012;59(1):511–8.
18. Mayer AR, Ling JM, Allen EA, et al. Static and dynamic intrinsic connectivity following mild traumatic brain injury. J Neurotrauma 2015;32(14):1046–55.
19. Sours C, Rosenberg J, Kane R, et al. Associations between interhemispheric functional connectivity and

the Automated Neuropsychological Assessment Metrics (ANAM) in civilian mild TBI. Brain Imaging Behav 2015;9(2):190–203.

20. Slobounov SM, Gay M, Zhang K, et al. Alteration of brain functional network at rest and in response to YMCA physical stress test in concussed athletes: RsFMRI study. Neuroimage 2011;55(4):1716–27.

21. Zhang K, Johnson B, Gay M, et al. Default mode network in concussed individuals in response to the YMCA physical stress test. J Neurotrauma 2012;29(5):756–65.

22. Wylie GR, Freeman K, Thomas A, et al. Cognitive improvement after mild traumatic brain injury measured with functional neuroimaging during the acute period. PLoS One 2015;10(5):e0126110.

23. Palacios EM, Yuh EL, Chang YS, et al. Resting-state functional connectivity alterations associated with six-month outcomes in mild traumatic brain injury. J Neurotrauma 2017;34(8):1546–57.

24. Young GR, Tsao JW. Rate of persistent postconcussive symptoms. JAMA 2017;317(13):1375.

25. Whitlow CT, Casanova R, Maldjian JA. Effect of resting-state fMRI-BOLD acquisition duration on stability of graph theory network metrics of brain network connectivity. Radiology 2011;259:516–24.

26. Zhou Y. Small world properties changes in mild traumatic brain injury. J Magn Reson Imaging 2016; 46(2):518–27.

27. Ellis MJ, Ryner LN, Sobczyk O, et al. Neuroimaging assessment of cerebrovascular reactivity in concussion: current concepts, methodological considerations, and review of the literature. Front Neurol 2016;7:1–16.

28. Adelson PD, Srinivas R, Chang Y, et al. Cerebrovascular response in children following severe traumatic brain injury. Childs Nerv Syst 2011;27:1465–76.

29. Xiong KL, Zhang JN, Zhang YL, et al. Brain functional connectivity and cognition in mild traumatic brain injury. Neuroradiology 2016;58(7):733–9.

30. Stevens MC, Lovejoy D, Kim J, et al. Multiple resting state network functional connectivity abnormalities in mild traumatic brain injury. Brain Imaging Behav 2012;6(2):293–318.

31. Posner MI, Rothbart MK, Sheese BE, et al. The anterior cingulate gyrus and the mechanism of self-regulation. Cogn Affect Behav Neurosci 2007; 7(4):391–5.

32. Zhou Y, Lui YW, Zuo XN, et al. Characterization of thalamo-cortical association using amplitude and connectivity of functional MRI in mild traumatic brain injury. J Magn Reson Imaging 2014;39(6): 1558–68.

33. Banks SD, Coronado RA, Clemons LR, et al. Thalamic functional connectivity in mild traumatic brain injury: longitudinal associations with patient-reported outcomes and neuropsychological tests. Arch Phys Med Rehabil 2016;97(8):1254–61.

34. Bharath RD, Munivenkatappa A, Gohel S, et al. Recovery of resting brain connectivity ensuing mild traumatic brain injury. Front Hum Neurosci 2015;9:513.

35. Iraji A, Chen H, Wiseman N, et al. Compensation through functional hyperconnectivity: a longitudinal connectome assessment of mild traumatic brain injury. Neural Plast 2016;2016:4072402.

36. Mayer AR, Mannell MV, Ling J, et al. Functional connectivity in mild traumatic brain injury. Hum Brain Mapp 2011;32(11):1825–35.

37. Sharp DJ, Beckmann CF, Greenwood R, et al. Default mode network functional and structural connectivity after traumatic brain injury. Brain 2011; 134(8):2233–47.

38. Tang L, Ge Y, Sodickson DK, et al. Thalamic resting-state functional networks: disruption in patients with mild traumatic brain injury. Radiology 2011;260(3): 831–40.

39. Westfall DR, West JD, Bailey JN, et al. Increased brain activation during working memory processing after pediatric mild traumatic brain injury (mTBI). J Pediatr Rehabil Med 2015;8(4):297–308.

40. Broglio S, Eckner J, Paulson H, et al. Cognitive decline and aging: the role of concussive and subconcussive impacts. Exerc Sport Sci Rev 2012; 40(3):138–44.

41. McKee A, Cantu R, Nowinski C, et al. Chronic traumatic encephalopathy in athletes: progressive tauopathy following repetitive head injury. J Neuropathol Exp Neurol 2009;68(7):709–35.

42. Orr CA, Albaugh MD, Watts R, et al. Neuroimaging biomarkers of a history of concussion observed in asymptomatic young athletes. J neurotrauma 2016; 33(9):803–10.

43. Gilmore CS, Camchong J, Davenport ND, et al. Deficits in visual system functional connectivity after blast-related mild TBI are associated with injury severity and executive dysfunction. Brain Behav 2016;6(5):e00454.

44. Vakhtin AA, Calhoun VD, Jung RE, et al. Changes in intrinsic functional brain networks following blast-induced mild traumatic brain injury. Brain Inj 2013; 27(11):1304–10.

45. Rangaprakash D, Deshpande G, Daniel TA, et al. Compromised hippocampus-striatum pathway as a potential imaging biomarker of mild-traumatic brain injury and posttraumatic stress disorder. Hum Brain Mapp 2017;38(6):2843–64.

46. Nordin LE, Möller MC, Julin P, et al. Post mTBI fatigue is associated with abnormal brain functional connectivity. Sci Rep 2016;6:21183.

Diffusion MR Imaging in Mild Traumatic Brain Injury

Maria J. Borja, MD[a],*, Sohae Chung, PhD[b],
Yvonne W. Lui, MD[a]

KEYWORDS

• DWI • Diffusion • MR imaging • Mild traumatic brain injury • Kurtosis • Advanced imaging

KEY POINTS

- Advanced diffusion-weighted MR imaging is of particular interest in the study of mild traumatic brain injury because changes in diffusion reflect underlying changes in microstructure.
- Diffusion-weighted imaging, diffusion tensor imaging, and diffusion kurtosis imaging can reveal alterations in the brain parenchyma in acute and chronic mTBI that are not identified with standard central nervous system imaging.
- Specific areas of the brain have shown vulnerability to damage after mild injury and may correlate with altered cognitive performance.
- Promising technical developments are being made and efforts are underway to pursue larger, multi-center trials with standardized methodology to better understand what detected changes in diffusion MR imaging represent.

INTRODUCTION

The term "mild" in mild traumatic brain injury (mTBI) greatly understates the significance of injury when considering its major implications to patients and society. Up to 30% of patients who have suffered mTBI do not recover in the first 3 months postinjury and may suffer long-term or permanent deficits.[1,2] It is estimated that 70% to 90% of all hospital-treated head injuries are mild, with an incidence of approximately 300 in 100,000[3]; however, the true incidence is likely higher considering that many patients with mild injuries are either not treated at hospitals or not treated at all.[2,3]

Early recognition of mTBI is important because prompt medical treatment and rehabilitation are believed to improve outcome.[1] Unfortunately, standard central nervous system imaging, such as computed tomography (CT) and conventional MR imaging, has limited sensitivity for mTBI, often failing to detect brain damage despite the presence of known injury.[1,2,4] This has motivated the search for imaging biomarkers of injury in this group of patients, particularly markers that reflect patient symptoms and predict patient outcome. One of the major known forms of parenchymal injury in mTBI is axonal injury,[1] which makes advanced diffusion-weighted (DWI) MR imaging of particular interest because changes in diffusion reflect underlying changes in microstructure. Over the past decade, much has been learned regarding diffusion MR imaging, mTBI, and the use of diffusion MR imaging to detect and evaluate injury in these patients.[1,2,5]

[a] Department of Radiology, New York University School of Medicine, 660 1st Avenue, New York, NY 10016, USA; [b] Department of Radiology, New York University School of Medicine, Center for Advanced Imaging Innovation and Research, Bernard and Irene Schwartz Center for Biomedical Imaging, 660 1st Avenue, New York, NY 10016, USA
* Corresponding author.
E-mail address: Maria.BorjaAngulo@nyumc.org

Neuroimag Clin N Am 28 (2018) 117–126
https://doi.org/10.1016/j.nic.2017.09.009
1052-5149/18/© 2017 Elsevier Inc. All rights reserved.

DIFFUSION-WEIGHTED IMAGING

Restricted diffusion (ie, reduced diffusivity) on DWI can be seen in several processes, most notably cytotoxic edema, which occurs when ischemia is associated with cellular edema, typically in acute infarction.[6] There are, however, other causes of cytotoxic edema, particularly excitotoxic edema. Excitotoxic edema is triggered by the release of a high concentration of glutamate, which then results in intramyelinic edema, a reversible cause of cytotoxic edema. Restricted diffusion may occur acutely after white matter injury[7] (**Fig. 1**), although the exact mechanism is still uncertain. Some of the proposed theories for the presence of transient restricted diffusion in traumatic axonal injury include the release of glutamate from injury,

resulting in excitotoxic edema[6]; the presence of associated hypoxia and hypotension, leading to trauma-induced ischemia[8]; or cytoskeletal collapse of the injured axons that would further hinder the motion of free water molecules.[9] In contrast, increased diffusivity is seen in the setting of increased extracellular water such as in with vasogenic edema.[1] Lesions from traumatic axonal injury, therefore, may show variable signal on DWI, depending on timing after injury and, because of the aforementioned mechanisms, may exhibit either increased or decreased diffusivity.[7]

Total number and volume of lesions on DWI (both with increased and decreased diffusivity) in the acute phase after head injury is shown to strongly correlate with memory deficits in mild trauma,[10] as well as with the modified Rankin Scale in

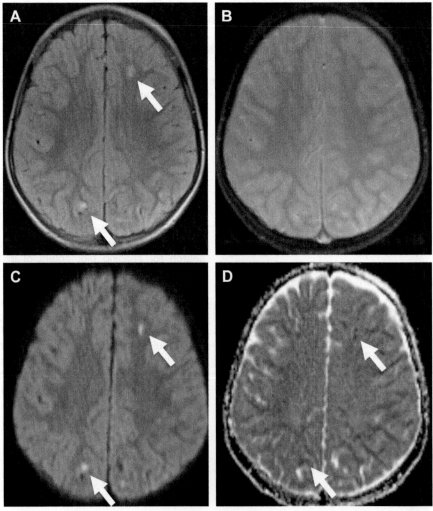

Fig. 1. A 5-year-old boy with traumatic axonal injury at the level of the centrum semiovale. The lesions (*arrows*) are hyperintense on fluid-attenuated inversion recovery (FLAIR) (*A*), do not demonstrate appreciate susceptibility on T2*-weighted images (*B*), and show restricted diffusion on DWI (*C*) and apparent diffusion coefficient maps (*D*), reflecting acute injury.

moderate to severe trauma.[7] Importantly, however, although DWI has proven to detect some additional lesions not evident on T2* or fluid-attenuated inversion recovery (FLAIR), its sensitivity for lesion detection remains limited because it may not depict all of the injuries seen on other sequences.[11]

DIFFUSION TENSOR IMAGING

Diffusion tensor imaging (DTI) is a diffusion MR imaging method that measures directional diffusion of water molecules in vivo and is, therefore, of particular interest in disorders of white matter. Notably, individual axons are not resolved using DTI. Instead, the generalized diffusion properties of a white matter fiber bundle can be depicted and, with that, information about the direction and course of WM bundles can be inferred.[2] Based on this principle, DTI can indirectly reveal changes to axonal microstructure after mTBI.[12]

FRACTIONAL ANISOTROPY

The main quantitative metric derived from DTI is fractional anisotropy (FA), a measure of anisotropic diffusion.[2] Higher FA is associated with homogeneity in fiber orientation, increased fiber density or axonal diameter, and increased ratio of intracellular or extracellular space.[4] Decreased white matter FA may occur due to a variety of histopathologic changes, including damage to myelin, damage to axon membranes, reduced number of axons, decreased axonal coherence, and increased edema.

Alterations in FA have been found in patients with mTBI in both acute (time from injury <2 weeks) and chronic phases. In the chronic phase after mTBI, most reports are consistent and reveal various areas of reduced FA.[1,5,13–15] Inglese and colleagues[16] reported reduced FA in multiple areas of the brain, including corpus callosum, internal capsule, and centrum semiovale, through grouped region of interest (ROI) analysis in 26 subjects with chronic mTBI. Studies by Salmond and colleagues,[17] Kraus and colleagues,[18] and Little and colleagues[19] evaluated 16, 20, and 12 subjects with chronic mTBI, respectively. They also found decreased FA in multiple regions of the brain using grouped voxel-based analysis, ROI, and histogram analysis. Both grouped and individual voxel-based analysis performed by Lipton and colleagues[20] on 17 subjects with chronic mTBI demonstrated similar reductions in FA.

The reported FA values in the acute phase after mTBI are variable. FA values may be increased and/or decreased.[5,13,14,16,20–27] Fig. 2 gives representative examples of the

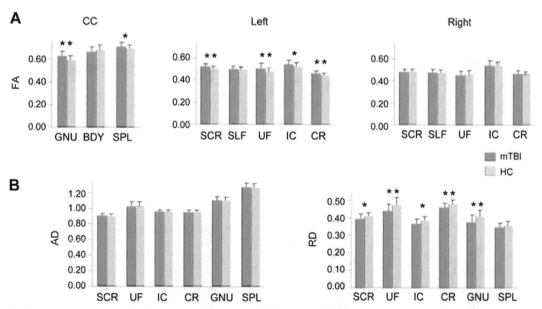

Fig. 2. Mean FA values (*A*) from ROI in the genu (GNU), body (BDY), and splenium (SPL) of the corpus callosum (CC), superior corona radiata (SCR), superior longitudinal fasciculus (SLF), uncinate fasciculus (UF), corona radiata (CR), and internal capsule (IC). Patients with mTBI (*green bars*) showed mostly higher FA values than healthy controls (*gray bars*). Significance is indicated with double asterisks, statistical trends with single asterisk. Axial diffusivity and radial diffusivity (*B*) measurements from mTBI patients and healthy controls for regions with statistical differences in FA. (*From* Mayer AR, Ling J, Mannell MV, et al. A prospective diffusion tensor imaging study in mild traumatic brain injury. Neurology 2010;74(8):643–50; with permission.)

differences in FA changes reported in the literature (Fig. 3). Several metaanalyses and reviews of the literature agree that both elevated and reduced FA can be seen in subjects in the acute phase of injury after mTBI.[1,4,5,13,15] In a 2014 metaanalysis of mTBI subjects, Eierud and colleagues[13] reviewed 122 publications reporting DTI results after mTBI over the past 21 years and concluded that increased FA in the acute phase was reported more frequently than decreased FA. This could be due to a variety of reasons, including axonal injury in areas of crossing fibers and significantly reduced extracellular diffusivity in the setting of cytotoxic edema.[1] Wilde and colleagues[4] demonstrated a more complex, heterogeneous pattern of anisotropy in which FA fluctuated in the acute stage. These investigators performed serial DTI in 8 subjects with mTBI at 4 different time points

within the first week after injury, noting acute transient increases of FA in the left cingulum bundle at variable time points.

Only a few longitudinal studies have been performed in subjects with mTBI.[14,27–31] These longitudinal data, though limited, corroborate the presence of variable changes in FA in brain parenchyma. Normalization, partial normalization, and worsening abnormal FA values compared with healthy controls have all been reported in longitudinal studies and may reflect tissue repair, partial tissue recovery, and continued tissue damage.[28] Mayer and colleagues[14] examined 15 healthy controls and 10 subjects in the semiacute stage after mTBI, 12 days after injury, and 3 to 5 months later. They found partial normalization of previously abnormal FA values in the splenium and corona radiata of subjects on follow-up. Arfanakis and colleagues[27] evaluated

A Significant cortical regions of interest

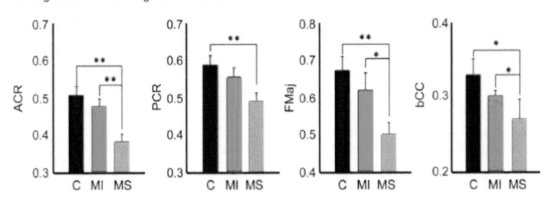

B Significant subcortical regions of interest

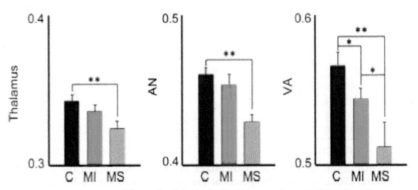

Fig. 3. Mean FA extracted from the (A) anterior corona radiata (ACR), posterior corona radiata (PCR), forceps major (fMaj), and body of the corpus callosum (bCC), as well as from the (B) thalamus, anterior thalamic nucleus (AN) and ventral anterior thalamic nucleus (VA). Patients with mTBI (MI) showed lower FA than controls (C), but higher than moderate/severe TBI (MS). Significance is indicated (*P = .05; **P = .01). (From Little DM, Kraus MF, Joseph J, et al. Thalamic integrity underlies executive dysfunction in traumatic brain injury. Neurology 2010;74(7):558–64; with permission.)

2 subjects 24 hours after injury and 1 month after injury and found partial and complete normalization of previously decreased FA values in several white matter regions on follow-up. In a longitudinal study on mTBI, Grossman and colleagues[28] studied 16 controls and 20 subjects with mTBI 1 month and 9 months after injury and reported variable changes in different brain regions for DTI, diffusion kurtosis imaging (DKI), and arterial spin labeling (ASL) measures with time. MacDonald and colleagues[29] studied 63 subjects from military personnel with mTBI within 90 days after injury and after 6 to 12 months for follow-up. Using ROIs in grouped and individual analysis compared with controls, regions of low FA were reported in the acute phase with partial normalization on the follow-up scans. Eighteen concussed athletes within 6 days and at 6 months after injury were evaluated by Henry and colleagues[31] using grouped voxel-based analysis. They observed higher FA, higher axial diffusivity (AD), and lower mean diffusivity (MD) values in the corpus callosum and corticospinal tracts of concussed subjects in the acute and chronic setting, without significant change between acute versus chronic stages.

AXIAL AND RADIAL DIFFUSIVITY

Other metrics that can be quantified using DTI data include AD and radial diffusivity (RD). AD refers to the magnitude of diffusion along the long axis of the fiber tract, thought to be affected by pathologic processes involving axons. RD refers to the diffusivity perpendicular to the fiber tract, thought to be affected by pathologic processes involving myelin.[1,2,15] These metrics have also been explored in an effort to improve the sensitivity of DTI to mTBI. FA, MD, AD, and RD are mutually related[13]; however, AD and RD show different patterns when assessing patients with traumatic brain injury (TBI) in terms of time since injury and severity of injury.[15] According to the current literature,[14,25] in the acute and subacute phase of mTBI, AD seems to remain comparable to that of controls, whereas RD has been reported to be both elevated[25] and reduced.[14] In the study by Kumar and colleagues,[25] elevated RD values were observed in the genu and splenium of 26 subjects with mTBI compared with 33 healthy controls, using ROI analysis in the acute period (within 5–14 days) after injury. In contrast, Mayer and colleagues[14] observed low RD in the genu and several left hemispheric white matter tracts in 22 subjects with mTBI, using ROI analysis during the acute

to subacute stages of trauma (within 21 days, mean of 12).

In the chronic phase after injury, Kraus and colleagues[18] found elevated AD values throughout all severities of trauma, whereas RD changes seemed to depend on injury severity. The investigators found no significant difference in RD in 20 subjects with mild chronic injury when compared with controls but higher RD in chronic moderate or severe TBI. These differences in RD are likely due to the intrinsic diversity of neuroinflammatory mechanisms in TBI[15] and possibly irreparable damage to myelin with greater degrees of injury.

DIFFUSION KURTOSIS IMAGING

The model used for DTI at typical maximal b-values of 1000 s/mm^2 is based on assuming a Gaussian distribution of diffusion. At higher b-values, however, diffusion displacement in white matter is known to be non-Gaussian. DKI uses multishell imaging with multiple b-values beyond 1000 to quantify this non-Gaussian behavior (Fig. 4).[32,33] Kurtosis is a measure of the deviation from a Gaussian distribution and is a measure of tissue microstructural complexity.[2,34] Thus, DKI has theoretic advantages in detecting subtle injury in tissue and may be of specific utility in areas normally shown to have relatively low FA in which the potential of DTI metrics to detect injury may be lower.

DKI results in the literature are consistent with DTI findings in longitudinal studies and may provide additional information about DTI.[28,35] In a longitudinal study by Grossman and colleagues,[28] 20 subjects with mTBI demonstrated significant differences from 16 controls in DTI, DKI, and ASL measures in the thalamus and

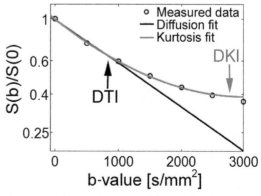

Fig. 4. Signal intensity versus diffusion b-value. Graph of signal intensity against diffusion b-value demonstrating improved modeling of DKI compared with DTI at higher b-values. S(b)/S(0), normalized signal.

white matter within 1 month and 9 months after injury, correlating with cognitive performance. **Fig. 5**, reprinted from this longitudinal study, illustrates differences in mean kurtosis (MK) in the thalamus of impaired and unimpaired subjects with mTBI compared with controls. Results show that impaired subjects with TBI had lower MK values than unimpaired subjects and controls (see **Fig. 5**). Reduced MK and radial kurtosis but no significant changes in DTI were reported in the anterior internal capsule of 24 subjects with mTBI when examined in a longitudinal study by Stokum and colleagues[35] at 10 days, 1 month, and 6 months postinjury. Improvements in cognition 1 to 6 months after injury correlated with changes in MK and radial kurtosis in the thalamus, internal capsule, and corpus callosum. Lancaster and colleagues[36] performed DTI and DKI in 26 high school and college athletes with sports-related concussion within 24 hours from injury and at 8 days. They found higher axial kurtosis in the corpus callosum and several white matter tracts in subjects compared with controls, which also positively correlated with symptoms.

INJURY LOCALIZATION

Despite variations in methodology, group analysis with DTI points to several specific anatomic regions of frequent injury in mTBI,[13] suggesting vulnerability of these areas.[2] Frequently reported areas of white matter injury include frontal lobe, corpus callosum, posterior limb of internal capsule, cingulum, and fronto-occipital fasciculus.[5,37] In addition to white

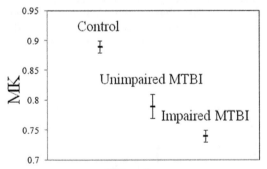

Thalamus

Fig. 5. Mean (*hash marks*) and standard error (*lines*) for thalamic mean kurtosis (MK) in controls, and for cognitively normal and cognitively impaired subjects. Cognitively impaired subjects show significantly lower MK in the thalamus than unimpaired subjects and controls. (*From* Grossman EJ, Jensen JH, Babb JS, et al. Cognitive impairment in mild traumatic brain injury: a longitudinal diffusional kurtosis and perfusion imaging study. AJNR Am J Neuroradiol 2013;34(5):951–7, 955; with permission.)

matter injury, thalamic injury has been described in mTBI.[19,37] Although this information is applicable for group analyses, reliably detecting specific areas of injury in individual subjects remains a work in progress.[38]

DIFFUSION TRACTOGRAPHY

Diffusion tractography relates diffusion profiles across voxels and reconstructs structural diffusion pathways in the brain corresponding to major visualized white matter fiber bundles.

Limitations include lack of standardization of tractography algorithms and potential low sensitivity for detecting small lesions.[15,39] Deterministic tractography, currently among the most popular methods of tractography available on vendor platforms, does not account for crossing fibers and tracts that have broad, multidimensional direction.[2] Research efforts to solve these problems include high angular resolution diffusion imaging (HARDI) and diffusion spectrum imaging (DSI).[1,15]

DIFFUSION AND COGNITION

Conventional imaging findings in mTBI do not correlate with neurocognitive performance. In contradistinction, the global burden of disease in mTBI measured by DTI (ie, number of DTI lesions detected or average FA over multiple ROIs) is reported to correlate with executive function and cognitive processing speed.[15] Miles and colleagues[26] studied 17 subjects with mTBI and found a positive correlation between low FA and poor executive function, as measured in the Prioritization Form B test. Results from a study of Niogi and colleagues[40] of 34 subjects with mTBI suggest negative correlation between overall number of DTI lesions (defined as FA <2.5 SD from the average in a set of predetermined ROIs) and the mean reaction time in the cognitive tasks performed (attention network task).

In addition to global burden of injury, current literature suggests that injuries in specific areas of the brain, such as frontal white matter, correlate with poor attention, memory, learning, and executive function.[13,28,41] Lipton and colleagues[41] reported a positive correlation between low FA in the frontal white matter and poor performance on tests of executive function (continuous performance task and the executive maze task) in 34 subjects with mTBI studied 2 to 14 days after the trauma. There is an increasing body of literature associating alterations of thalamic diffusion with altered neuropsychological studies in mTBI.[37] Little and colleagues[19] found a correlation between low thalamic FA and lower scores on neurocognitive tests of attention, memory, and executive function performed in 12 subjects with mTBI within 12 months from the injury. A DKI study performed by Grossman and colleagues[37] evaluating 20 subjects with mTBI, also demonstrated lower MK and FA in the thalamus and internal capsule of subjects with cognitive impairment compared with subjects without cognitive impairment, within and after 1 year from mild trauma.

Altered performance in neuropsychological tests may variably correlate with FA values. In a metaanalysis of mTBI, Eierud and colleagues[13] found poor neuropsychological performance correlated with high FA in the acute phase and low FA in the chronic phase. Others; for example, Wilde and colleagues,[4] studied 8 subjects with mTBI within 8 days postinjury and found inconsistent correlation between FA values and performance on memory tasks. The pattern of FA was variable (sometimes transiently elevated), independent of the task performance.

SPECIAL POPULATIONS: PEDIATRIC PATIENTS

Children, age 0 to 4 years, and adolescents, age 15 to 19, are at high risk for TBI,[28,42] though they are less likely to report postconcussive symptoms and have better outcomes than older patients, possibly due to greater neuroplasticity.[43,44] Despite being a high-risk group for head injury, few studies specifically address the pediatric population.[21,24,45] The available studies mirror some of the results derived from adult data with elevated FA, decreased MD, and decreased RD in the acute phase involving corpus callosum and cingulum bundle.[21,24,45]

Changes in FA and RD in adolescents with mTBI have also been reported to correlate with both performance on neuropsychological tests and postconcussive symptoms.[21,45] A DTI study by Wu and colleagues[45] on 12 adolescents (range 14–17 years) 1 to 6 days post-mTBI showed a correlation between high FA in the left cingulum bundle with poor episodic verbal learning and memory task. Wilde and colleagues[21] performed DTI in the corpus callosum of 10 adolescents with mTBI 1 to 6 days after trauma and found that increased FA and decreased RD in the corpus callosum correlates with the severity of postconcussion symptoms. High FA in the frontal and supracallosal white matter was also found in the chronic stage of mTBI 6 to 12 months postinjury in 24 subjects of ages 10 to 18 years, compared with 24 controls in a study performed by Wozniak and colleagues.[46]

To the authors' knowledge, there are no current published studies using DKI in pediatric patients with mTBI.

SEX DIFFERENCES

The impact of sex and progesterone on TBI risk, severity, and outcome remains a controversy, in view of the limited literature and conflicting results. Several studies using neuropsychological testing and symptom scale questionnaires[44,47–49] suggest women may have worse outcome compared with men. Contrary to some of the existing literature, a DTI study of mTBI subjects by Fakhran and colleagues[50] concluded that male sex was an independent risk factor for persistent postconcussive symptoms at 3 months after injury. In addition, a Cochrane review of the literature, including 8 studies that investigated the effects of progesterone in TBI, did not find sufficient evidence to prove that progesterone could reduce mortality or disability in subjects with TBI.[51]

ONGOING RESEARCH

Creation of a normative atlas is considered a fundamental step in the future of mTBI imaging research, which would allow the establishment of normative values and an accurate comparison between subjects and healthy subjects.[12]

Efforts are underway to pursue larger, multicenter trials with standardized methodology. The National Institute of Neurologic Disorders and Stroke (NINDS)-funded, multicenter Transforming Research and Clinical Knowledge in Traumatic Brain Injury (TRACK-TBI) study aims to collect and analyze detailed clinical data on 3000 subjects at 11 US sites, across the injury spectrum, along with CT or MR imaging, blood biospecimens, and detailed clinical outcomes (https://tracktbi. ucsf.edu). The TRACK-TBI Pilot dataset is the first to populate the Federal Interagency Traumatic Brain Injury Research (FITBIR) repository and, with the current TRACK-TBI data, is compatible with the International Initiative for Traumatic Brain Injury Research (InTBIR), a collaborative effort of the European Commission (EC), the Canadian Institutes of Health Research (CIHR) and the National Institutes of Health (NIH). The Federal Interagency TBI Research (FITBIR) Informatics System (https://fitbir.nih.gov/) is the result of a collaboration that began in 2011 between the NIH and the US Department of Defense. Its purpose is to create a national resource for archiving and sharing clinical data from research studies on TBI, along with appropriate control data.[38]

Efforts to improve sensitivity and specificity of diffusion MR imaging for detecting injury in mTBI[12] are ongoing. Promising technical developments are being made on acquisition and postprocessing, as well as modeling. Multidimensional, multishell

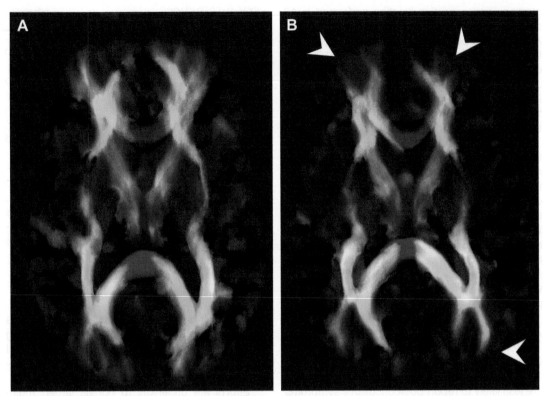

Fig. 6. Directionally encoded color track-density imaging maps in a 37-year-old man with mTBI (*B*) and a healthy control matched for age and sex (*A*) show global relative paucity of peripheral tracts extending to the subcortical region (*arrowheads*) compared with the healthy control.

acquisitions, such as HARDI and DSI, allow for resolution of crossing fibers by measuring intravoxel diffusion in multiple directions.[52] Multitensor models allow tracing of small, peripheral fiber bundles.[53] Track-density imaging is a postprocessing technique using super resolution to obtain intravoxel information derived by whole-brain probabilistic streamline tractography.[54] This allows for visualization of smaller pathways that are typically not identified using conventional DTI and can work toward solving the problem of crossing fibers (Fig. 6).[55]

Newer, quantitative analyses use compartment-specific modeling of diffusion in both intracellular and extracellular spaces. This allows the derivation of modeled metrics believed to have greater biophysical meaning than traditional empirical DTI and DKI metrics. Such modeled metrics include axonal water fraction (a marker of axon density),[56] intraaxonal diffusivity (a marker of intra-axonal injury),[57] extraaxonal axial and radial diffusivities (eg, markers of changes in extraaxonal space associated with gliosis, astrocytosis, extracellular inflammation), and extraaxonal tortuosity (a marker of myelination or alignment of fibers).[58] Extraaxonal RD would also be sensitive to demyelination.[56] These newer metrics provide more

information beyond the traditional empiric diffusion metrics such as FA.

SUMMARY

Remarkable advances have been made in the last decade in the use of diffusion MR imaging to study mTBI.[1,2,5,13] Diffusion shows differences between mTBI subjects and healthy control groups in multiple different metrics using a variety of techniques, supporting the notion that there are microstructural injuries in mTBI patients that radiologists have previously been insensitive to.

Important future areas of discovery in diffusion MR imaging and mTBI include larger longitudinal studies to improve the understanding of the evolution of injury after mTBI and unravel the biophysical meaning of what detected changes in diffusion MR imaging may represent.

REFERENCES

1. Grossman EJ, Inglese M, Bammer R. Mild traumatic brain injury: is diffusion imaging ready for primetime in forensic medicine? Top Magn Reson Imaging 2010;21(6):379–86.

2. Shenton ME, Hamoda HM, Schneiderman JS, et al. A review of magnetic resonance imaging and diffusion tensor imaging findings in mild traumatic brain injury. Brain Imaging Behav 2012;6(2):137–92.

3. Cassidy JD, Carroll LJ, Peloso PM, et al. Incidence, risk factors and prevention of mild traumatic brain injury: results of the WHO Collaborating Centre Task Force on Mild Traumatic Brain Injury. J Rehabil Med 2004;(43 Suppl):28–60.

4. Wilde EA, McCauley SR, Barnes A, et al. Serial measurement of memory and diffusion tensor imaging changes within the first week following uncomplicated mild traumatic brain injury. Brain Imaging Behav 2012;6(2):319–28.

5. Hulkower MB, Poliak DB, Rosenbaum SB, et al. A decade of DTI in traumatic brain injury: 10 years and 100 articles later. AJNR Am J Neuroradiol 2013;34(11):2064–74.

6. Al Brashdi YH, Albayram MS. Reversible restricted-diffusion lesion representing transient intramyelinic cytotoxic edema in a patient with traumatic brain injury. Neuroradiol J 2015;28(4):409–12.

7. Schaefer PW, Huisman TA, Sorensen AG, et al. Diffusion-weighted MR imaging in closed head injury: high correlation with initial Glasgow coma scale score and score on modified Rankin scale at discharge. Radiology 2004;233(1):58–66.

8. Ito J, Marmarou A, Barzo P, et al. Characterization of edema by diffusion-weighted imaging in experimental traumatic brain injury. J Neurosurg 1996; 84(1):97–103.

9. Povlishock JT, Christman CW. The pathobiology of traumatically induced axonal injury in animals and humans: a review of current thoughts. J Neurotrauma 1995;12(4):555–64.

10. Kurca E, Sivak S, Kucera P. Impaired cognitive functions in mild traumatic brain injury patients with normal and pathologic magnetic resonance imaging. Neuroradiology 2006;48(9):661–9.

11. Ezaki Y, Tsutsumi K, Morikawa M, et al. Role of diffusion-weighted magnetic resonance imaging in diffuse axonal injury. Acta Radiol 2006;47(7): 733–40.

12. Koerte IK, Hufschmidt J, Muehlmann M, et al. Advanced neuroimaging of mild traumatic brain injury. In: Laskowitz D, Grant G, editors. Translational research in traumatic brain injury. Boca Raton (FL): CRC Press; 2016. p. 277–98.

13. Eierud C, Craddock RC, Fletcher S, et al. Neuroimaging after mild traumatic brain injury: review and meta-analysis. Neuroimage Clin 2014;4:283–94.

14. Mayer AR, Ling J, Mannell MV, et al. A prospective diffusion tensor imaging study in mild traumatic brain injury. Neurology 2010;74(8):643–50.

15. Niogi SN, Mukherjee P. Diffusion tensor imaging of mild traumatic brain injury. J Head Trauma Rehabil 2010;25(4):241–55.

16. Inglese M, Makani S, Johnson G, et al. Diffuse axonal injury in mild traumatic brain injury: a diffusion tensor imaging study. J Neurosurg 2005; 103(2):298–303.

17. Salmond CH, Menon DK, Chatfield DA, et al. Diffusion tensor imaging in chronic head injury survivors: correlations with learning and memory indices. Neuroimage 2006;29(1):117–24.

18. Kraus MF, Susmaras T, Caughlin BP, et al. White matter integrity and cognition in chronic traumatic brain injury: a diffusion tensor imaging study. Brain 2007;130(Pt 10):2508–19.

19. Little DM, Kraus MF, Joseph J, et al. Thalamic integrity underlies executive dysfunction in traumatic brain injury. Neurology 2010;74(7):558–64.

20. Lipton ML, Gellella E, Lo C, et al. Multifocal white matter ultrastructural abnormalities in mild traumatic brain injury with cognitive disability: a voxel-wise analysis of diffusion tensor imaging. J Neurotrauma 2008;25(11):1335–42.

21. Wilde EA, McCauley SR, Hunter JV, et al. Diffusion tensor imaging of acute mild traumatic brain injury in adolescents. Neurology 2008;70(12):948–55.

22. Bazarian JJ, Zhong J, Blyth B, et al. Diffusion tensor imaging detects clinically important axonal damage after mild traumatic brain injury: a pilot study. J Neurotrauma 2007;24(9):1447–59.

23. Yallampalli R, Wilde EA, Bigler ED, et al. Acute white matter differences in the fornix following mild traumatic brain injury using diffusion tensor imaging. J Neuroimaging 2013;23(2):224–7.

24. Chu Z, Wilde EA, Hunter JV, et al. Voxel-based analysis of diffusion tensor imaging in mild traumatic brain injury in adolescents. AJNR Am J Neuroradiol 2010;31(2):340–6.

25. Kumar R, Gupta RK, Husain M, et al. Comparative evaluation of corpus callosum DTI metrics in acute mild and moderate traumatic brain injury: its correlation with neuropsychometric tests. Brain Inj 2009; 23(7):675–85.

26. Miles L, Grossman RI, Johnson G, et al. Short-term DTI predictors of cognitive dysfunction in mild traumatic brain injury. Brain Inj 2008;22(2):115–22.

27. Arfanakis K, Haughton VM, Carew JD, et al. Diffusion tensor MR imaging in diffuse axonal injury. AJNR Am J Neuroradiol 2002;23(5):794–802.

28. Grossman EJ, Jensen JH, Babb JS, et al. Cognitive impairment in mild traumatic brain injury: a longitudinal diffusional kurtosis and perfusion imaging study. AJNR Am J Neuroradiol 2013;34(5):951–7. S951–3.

29. Mac Donald CL, Johnson AM, Cooper D, et al. Detection of blast-related traumatic brain injury in U.S. military personnel. N Engl J Med 2011; 364(22):2091–100.

30. Messe A, Caplain S, Paradot G, et al. Diffusion tensor imaging and white matter lesions at the subacute stage in mild traumatic brain injury with

persistent neurobehavioral impairment. Hum Brain Mapp 2011;32(6):999–1011.

31. Henry LC, Tremblay J, Tremblay S, et al. Acute and chronic changes in diffusivity measures after sports concussion. J Neurotrauma 2011;28(10):2049–59.

32. Jensen JH, Helpern JA. MRI quantification of non-Gaussian water diffusion by kurtosis analysis. NMR Biomed 2010;23(7):698–710.

33. Wintermark M, Sanelli PC, Anzai Y, et al, American College of Radiology Head Injury Institute. Imaging evidence and recommendations for traumatic brain injury: advanced neuro- and neurovascular imaging techniques. AJNR Am J Neuroradiol 2015;36(2):E1–11.

34. Fieremans E, Jensen JH, Helpern JA. White matter characterization with diffusional kurtosis imaging. Neuroimage 2011;58(1):177–88.

35. Stokum JA, Sours C, Zhuo J, et al. A longitudinal evaluation of diffusion kurtosis imaging in patients with mild traumatic brain injury. Brain Inj 2015; 29(1):47–57.

36. Lancaster MA, Olson DV, McCrea MA, et al. Acute white matter changes following sport-related concussion: a serial diffusion tensor and diffusion kurtosis tensor imaging study. Hum Brain Mapp 2016;37(11):3821–34.

37. Grossman EJ, Ge Y, Jensen JH, et al. Thalamus and cognitive impairment in mild traumatic brain injury: a diffusional kurtosis imaging study. J Neurotrauma 2012;29(13):2318–27.

38. Wintermark M, Coombs L, Druzgal TJ, et al. Traumatic brain injury imaging research roadmap. AJNR Am J Neuroradiol 2015;36(3):E12–23.

39. Gardner A, Kay-Lambkin F, Stanwell P, et al. A systematic review of diffusion tensor imaging findings in sports-related concussion. J Neurotrauma 2012;29(16):2521–38.

40. Niogi SN, Mukherjee P, Ghajar J, et al. Extent of microstructural white matter injury in postconcussive syndrome correlates with impaired cognitive reaction time: a 3T diffusion tensor imaging study of mild traumatic brain injury. AJNR Am J Neuroradiol 2008;29(5):967–73.

41. Lipton ML, Gulko E, Zimmerman ME, et al. Diffusion-tensor imaging implicates prefrontal axonal injury in executive function impairment following very mild traumatic brain injury. Radiology 2009;252(3):816–24.

42. Langlois JA, Rutland-Brown W, Wald MM. The epidemiology and impact of traumatic brain injury: a brief overview. J Head Trauma Rehabil 2006; 21(5):375–8.

43. Necajauskaite O, Endziniene M, Jureniene K. The prevalence, course and clinical features of postconcussion syndrome in children. Medicina (Kaunas) 2005;41(6):457–64.

44. Preiss-Farzanegan SJ, Chapman B, Wong TM, et al. The relationship between gender and postconcussion symptoms after sport-related mild traumatic brain injury. PM R 2009;1(3):245–53.

45. Wu TC, Wilde EA, Bigler ED, et al. Evaluating the relationship between memory functioning and cingulum bundles in acute mild traumatic brain injury using diffusion tensor imaging. J Neurotrauma 2010;27(2):303–7.

46. Wozniak JR, Krach L, Ward E, et al. Neurocognitive and neuroimaging correlates of pediatric traumatic brain injury: a diffusion tensor imaging (DTI) study. Arch Clin Neuropsychol 2007;22(5):555–68.

47. Ponsford J, Willmott C, Rothwell A, et al. Factors influencing outcome following mild traumatic brain injury in adults. J Int Neuropsychol Soc 2000;6(5):568–79.

48. Farace E, Alves WM. Do women fare worse: a meta-analysis of gender differences in traumatic brain injury outcome. J Neurosurg 2000;93(4):539–45.

49. Bazarian JJ, Blyth B, Mookerjee S, et al. Sex differences in outcome after mild traumatic brain injury. J Neurotrauma 2010;27(3):527–39.

50. Fakhran S, Yaeger K, Collins M, et al. Sex differences in white matter abnormalities after mild traumatic brain injury: localization and correlation with outcome. Radiology 2014;272(3):815–23.

51. Ma J, Huang S, Qin S, et al. Progesterone for acute traumatic brain injury. Cochrane Database Syst Rev 2012;(10):CD008409.

52. O'Donnell LJ, Westin CF. An introduction to diffusion tensor image analysis. Neurosurg Clin N Am 2011; 22(2):185–96, viii.

53. Malcolm JG, Shenton ME, Rathi Y. Filtered multitensor tractography. IEEE Trans Med Imaging 2010; 29(9):1664–75.

54. Calamante F, Tournier JD, Jackson GD, et al. Track-density imaging (TDI): super-resolution white matter imaging using whole-brain track-density mapping. Neuroimage 2010;53(4):1233–43.

55. Hoch MC, Chung S, Fatterpekar GM, et al. Track density imaging of hypertrophic olivary degeneration from multiple sclerosis plaque. BJR Case Rep 2016;2(4):20150299.

56. Jelescu IO, Zurek M, Winters KV, et al. In vivo quantification of demyelination and recovery using compartment-specific diffusion MRI metrics validated by electron microscopy. Neuroimage 2016;132:104–14.

57. Grossman EJ, Kirov II, Gonen O, et al. N-acetyl-aspartate levels correlate with intra-axonal compartment parameters from diffusion MRI. Neuroimage 2015;118:334–43.

58. Jelescu IO, Veraart J, Adisetiyo V, et al. One diffusion acquisition and different white matter models: how does microstructure change in human early development based on WMTI and NODDI? Neuroimage 2015;107:242–56.

Imaging of Chronic Concussion

Eliana Bonfante, MD*, Roy Riascos, MD, Octavio Arevalo, MD

KEYWORDS

- Concussion • Mild traumatic brain injury (mTBI) • Cerebral • Trauma
- Chronic traumatic encephalopathy (CTE)

KEY POINTS

- Cerebral concussion is a subset of traumatic brain injury resulting in transient impairment of neurologic function that usually resolves spontaneously, although in some cases, symptoms may be prolonged.
- Chronic traumatic encephalopathy is a recognized pathologic entity resulting from repetitive mild traumatic brain injury, clinically associated with progressive changes in memory, executive functioning, emotion and impulse control, and parkinsonism.
- CT and MR Imaging are the recommended imaging modalities to study patients with cerebral concussion. Although advanced neuroimaging techniques have shown significant potential to identify further injury and determine prognosis, their clinical utility is still under research.
- Conventional imaging findings in patients with cerebral concussion and chronic traumatic encephalopathy are absent or subtle in the majority of cases.
- The most common abnormalities include cerebral volume loss, enlargement of the cavum of the septum pellucidum, cerebral microhemorrhages, and white matter signal abnormalities, all of which have poor sensitivity and specificity.

GENERAL CONCEPTS

Cerebral concussion is a subset of traumatic brain injury (TBI) for which multiple definitions have been proposed. Some investigators use the terms, concussion and mild TBI (mTBI), interchangeably. The consensus statement from the 4th International Conference on Concussion in Sport, held in Zurich in November 2012, defined concussion as a brain injury and complex pathophysiologic process affecting the brain, induced by biomechanical forces. Common features in defining the nature of concussion include the following: (1) concussion may be caused either by a direct blow to the head, face, neck, or elsewhere on the body with an "impulsive" force transmitted to the head; (2) concussion typically results in the rapid onset of short-lived impairment of neurologic function that resolves spontaneously; in some cases, however, symptoms and signs may evolve over several minutes to hours; (3) concussion may result in neuropathological changes, but the acute clinical symptoms largely reflect a functional disturbance rather than a structural injury and, as such, no abnormality is seen on standard structural neuroimaging studies; and (4) concussion results in a graded set of clinical symptoms that may or may not involve loss of consciousness. Resolution of the clinical and cognitive symptoms typically follows a sequential course. In some cases, however, symptoms may be prolonged.[1]

The authors do not have any commercial or financial conflicts of interest and have no funding sources to disclose for the current project.
Department of Diagnostic and Interventional Imaging, The University of Texas Health Science Center at Houston, McGovern Medical School, 6431 Fannin Street MSB 2130B, Houston, TX 77030, USA
* Corresponding author.
E-mail address: Eliana.e.bonfante.mejia@uth.tmc.edu

neuroimaging.theclinics.com

Chronic traumatic encephalopathy (CTE), also denominated "dementia pugilistica," "punch drunk," or "boxer's dementia," was originally described in boxers and more recently associated with repetitive concussions in other sports (eg, American football). CTE is associated with progressive changes in memory, executive functioning, emotion (in particular depression), and impulse control as well as parkinsonism, with evidence for a distinction between syndromes dominated by mood and behavior (earlier onset) versus cognitive impairment (later onset, determined retrospectively). CTE has been observed as early as the late teenage years. In professional athletes, symptoms of CTE are typically seen 8 years to 10 years after an individual retires from play.[2] After neuropathologist Omalu and colleagues' publication in 2005,[3] raising an alert about the potential neuropathologic sequelae of repeated mTBI in professional football players, a strong reaction in the sports and medical communities triggered intense research in this field.

PATHOLOGIC STUDIES IN CHRONIC TRAUMATIC ENCEPHALOPATHY

In 2015 McKee and colleagues[4] conducted a postmortem evaluation of the brain of from a cohort of 85 subjects with histories of repetitive mTBI, including athletes and military veterans, and found evidence of CTE in 68 subjects.[4] The investigators described 4 stages in the progression of CTE.

Stage I was characterized by perivascular hyperphosphorylated tau (p-tau) neurofibrillary tangles in focal epicenters at the depths of the sulci in the superior, superior lateral, or inferior frontal cortex and was clinically associated with headache and loss of attention and concentration.

In stage II CTE, neurofibrillary tangles were found in superficial cortical layers adjacent to the focal epicenters and in the nucleus basalis of Meynert and locus coeruleus. Individuals with stage II CTE experienced depression and mood swings, explosivity, loss of attention and concentration, headache, and short-term memory loss.

Stage III CTE showed macroscopic evidence of mild cerebral atrophy, septal abnormalities, ventricular dilation, a sharply concave contour of the third ventricle and depigmentation of the locus coeruleus and substantia nigra. There was dense p-tau pathology in medial temporal lobe structures (hippocampus, entorhinal cortex, and amygdala) and widespread regions of the frontal, septal, temporal, parietal and insular cortices, diencephalon, brainstem, and spinal cord. Most individuals with stage III CTE demonstrated cognitive impairment with memory loss, executive dysfunction, loss of

attention and concentration, depression, explosivity, and visuospatial abnormalities.

Stage IV CTE was associated with further cerebral, medial temporal lobe, hypothalamic, thalamic and mammillary body atrophy, septal abnormalities, ventricular dilation, and pallor of the substantia nigra and locus coeruleus. Microscopically, p-tau pathology involved widespread regions of the neuraxis, including white matter, with prominent neuronal loss and gliosis of the cerebral cortex and hippocampal sclerosis. Subjects with stage IV CTE were uniformly demented with profound short-term memory loss, executive dysfunction, attention and concentration loss, explosivity, and aggression. Most also showed paranoia, depression, impulsivity, and visuospatial abnormalities. Advancing pathologic stage was associated with a significant decrease in brain weight and increased severity of cognitive abnormalities, supporting the validity of the pathologic staging scheme. In addition, pathologic stage correlated with duration of exposure to American football, survival after football, and age at death in those who played football.

In 2015, the neuropathologic criteria for diagnosis of CTE were refined by a panel of expert neuropathologists organized by the National Institute of Neurological Disorders and Stroke (NINDS) and the National Institute of Biomedical Imaging and Bioengineering. These criteria, presented in **Box 1**, have been used in subsequent pathology studies.[5]

In a review of more than 100 articles from both basic science and clinical medical literature, Giza and Hovda[6] described the pathophysiologic cascade after concussive brain injury. Experimental brain injury studies have shown acute abnormalities, including ionic fluxes, indiscriminate glutamate release, hyperglycolysis, lactate accumulation, and axonal injury. Later steps in this physiologic cascade involve increased intracellular calcium, mitochondrial dysfunction, impaired oxidative metabolism, decreased glycolysis, diminished cerebral blood flow, axonal disconnection, neurotransmitter disturbances, and delayed cell death. It is during this postinjury period, when cellular metabolism is already stretched to its limits, that the cell is more vulnerable to further insults.

EVIDENCE OF GLIAL DAMAGE

Kou and colleagues[7] described the glial damage in TBI. When TBI occurs, quiescent glia of multiple types become rapidly activated in a process termed, *reactive gliosis*. This process involves activated microglia initiating and sustaining astrocytic

Preliminary NINDS criteria for the pathologic diagnosis of chronic traumatic encephalopathy

Required for diagnosis of CTE

1. The pathognomonic lesion consists of p-tau aggregates in neurons, astrocytes, and cell processes around small vessels in an irregular pattern at the depths of the cortical sulci.

Supportive neuropathologic features of CTE

p-Tau–related pathologies

1. Abnormal p-tau immunoreactive pretangles and neurofibrillary tangles preferentially affecting superficial layers (layers II–III), in contrast to layers III and V as in AD

2. In the hippocampus, pretangles, neurofibrillary tangles, or extracellular tangles preferentially affecting CA2 and pretangles and prominent proximal dendritic swellings in CA4. These regional p-tau pathologies differ from the preferential involvement of CA1 and subiculum found in AD.

3. Abnormal p-tau immunoreactive neuronal and astrocytic aggregates in subcortical nuclei, including the mammillary bodies and other hypothalamic nuclei, amygdala, nucleus accumbens, thalamus, midbrain tegmentum, and isodendritic core (nucleus basalis of Meynert, raphe nuclei, substantia nigra, and locus coeruleus).

4. p-Tau immunoreactive thorny astrocytes at the glial limitans most commonly found in the subpial and periventricular regions

5. p-Tau immunoreactive large grainlike and dotlike structures (in addition to some threadlike neurites)

Non–p-tau–related pathologies

1. Macroscopic features: disproportionate dilatation of the third ventricle, septal abnormalities, mammillary body atrophy, and contusions or other signs of previous traumatic injury

2. TDP-43 immunoreactive neuronal cytoplasmic inclusions and dotlike structures in the hippocampus, anteromedial temporal cortex, and amygdala

Age-related p-tau astrogliopathy that may be present; nondiagnostic and nonsupportive

1. Patches of thorn-shaped astrocytes in subcortical white matter

2. Subependymal, periventricular, and perivascular thorn-shaped astrocytes in the mediobasal regions

3. Thorn-shaped astrocytes in amygdala or hippocampus

activation through the production and release of inflammatory mediators that in turn act on surrounding glia and neurons. This acute inflammatory process after the initial insult can function to regulate both degenerative and reparative events in the injured and recovering brain. Glial activation causes morphologic and functional changes within the cells, which effect the neural-glial and glial-glial interactions. This response can cause dysfunction of synaptic connections, imbalances of neurotransmitter homeostasis, and potential axonal degeneration and neuronal death. Historically, chronic neuroinflammation had been associated with neurologic diseases, such as multiple sclerosis, instead of injury. Several reports are linking single and repeated TBI events to chronic white matter outcomes associated with neuroinflammation. Neuropathology in preclinical and clinical studies has provided evidence that glial cells are a central component to the chronic white matter degenerative process.

RELATION OF CHRONIC TRAUMATIC ENCEPHALOPATHY AND NEURODEGENERATIVE DISORDERS

The link between chronic traumatic encephalopathy and neurodegenerative disorders, such as Parkinson disease, Alzheimer's disease (AD), Lewy body dementia, and frontotemporal dementia, has been examined by multiple investigators.[8–10] McKee and colleagues[4] noted that CTE appears distinguishable pathologically from other neurodegenerative diseases, especially with respect to topographic dispersion and, to a lesser degree, type of pathologic entity, and course (for example, slower rate of progression through stages).[4] Washington and colleagues[11] support the emergent theory that instead of considering TBI a risk factor for the precipitation of individual neurodegenerative diseases, TBI-induced neurodegenerative disease, or traumatic encephalopathy, is a spectrum disorder that shares clinical and neuropathological hallmarks with other neurodegenerative disorders.

Esopenko and colleagues[2] reviewed the literature on neurodegenerative disorders linked to remote TBI. The gross neuropathology of CTE is characterized by global volume reduction and ventricular enlargement; callosal thinning; atrophy in the medial temporal lobes, mammillary bodies, and brainstem; fenestrated cavum septum pellucidum (CSP); and scarring and neuronal loss of the cerebellar tonsils.

In a postmortem study of 52 subjects with TBI, with survivals ranging from 10 hours to 47 years postinjury, and 44 age-matched uninjured control subjects, selected from the Glasgow Traumatic Brain Injury Archive, Johnson and colleagues[12] attempted to characterize the neuroinflammatory response to brain injury, its temporal dynamics, and any potential role in neurodegeneration. The investigators found that with survival of greater than or equal to 3 months from injury, cases of TBI frequently displayed extensive, densely packed, reactive microglia (CR3/43-immunoreactive and/or CD68-immunoreactive), a pathology not seen in control subjects or acutely injured cases. These reactive microglia were present in 28% of cases with survival of greater than 1 year and up to 18 years posttrauma. In cases displaying this inflammatory pathology, evidence of ongoing white matter degradation could also be observed. Moreover, there was a 25% reduction in the corpus callosum thickness with survival greater than 1 year postinjury. These data present striking evidence of persistent inflammation and ongoing white matter degeneration for many years after just a single TBI in humans.

Evidence suggests that participation in contact–collision sports may increase the risk of neurodegenerative disorders, such as AD, but the data are conflicting.[13] Genetic factors, such as apolipoprotein E4, which has been studied in AD, may also be a risk factor for CTE.[14]

IMAGING FINDINGS

The guidelines of the American College of Radiology Head Injury Institute recommend noncontrast CT as the first line of imaging for patients with TBI and MR imaging in specific settings. Advanced neuroimaging techniques, including MR imaging–diffusion tensor imaging (DTI), blood oxygen level–dependent functional MR imaging, MR spectroscopy, perfusion imaging, PET/ single-photon emission CT (SPECT), and magnetoencephalography, are of particular interest in identifying further injury in patients with TBI when conventional CT and MR imaging findings are normal as well as for prognostication in patients with persistent symptoms.[15]

Evidence of parenchymal damage in CT is predictive of a poor functional outcome, as concluded by Smits and colleagues[16] in a study that included 237/312 patients with mTBI from the CT in Head Injury Patients study. The investigators assessed the association between CT findings and outcome using univariable and multivariable regression analysis. The Glasgow Outcome Scale was assessed at an average of 15 months after injury. Other outcome measures were the Modified Rankin Scale, the Barthel Index, and number and severity of postconcussive symptoms. There was

full recovery in 150 patients (63%), moderate disability in 70 (30%), severe disability in 7 (3.0%), and death in 10 (4.2%). Outcome according to the Modified Rankin Scale and Barthel Index was also favorable in most patients, but 82% of patients had postconcussive symptoms. Evidence of parenchymal damage (contusion or diffuse axonal injury) was the only independent predictor of poor functional outcome.

Conventional MR imaging sequences show structural changes, such as mass effect, midline shift, cisternal compression, internal loculations, or septations for subdural hematomas, blood in the contours of sulci and cisterns for subarachnoid hemorrhage, and volume changes for chronic postinjury analysis, such as hippocampal atrophy. Thin-slice 2-D or contiguous 3-D, T1-weighted and T2-weighted MR imaging offers high-resolution structural information for diagnosis, potential neurosurgical intervention, and volume quantification. A potentially useful quantitative marker of tissue damage is lesion load or total lesion volume.[17]

Parenchymal Volume Loss

Numerous studies have analyzed the relationship between TBI and parenchymal volume loss. Longitudinal studies (in which data are collected on more than 1 point in time) may be preferable to cross-sectional studies (1 point in time) for understanding the progression of brain atrophy after injury and understanding its association with important clinical variables. Ross[18] reviewed 10 longitudinal studies that measured volume loss in patients with TBI and found a consistent pattern of brain atrophy, which progressed over the months after injury. Atrophy correlated significantly with important clinical variables, such as loss of consciousness, duration of coma, duration of posttraumatic amnesia, hypoperfusion seen on acute SPECT, brain oxidative metabolism, and cerebral lactate-pyruvate ratio.

In a longitudinal study of 14 subjects with mild or moderate TBI and comparable controls, using a quantitative analysis of volume of brain parenchyma, MacKenzie and colleagues[19] concluded that whole-brain atrophy occurs after mild or moderate TBI and is evident at an average of 11 months after trauma. Injury that produces loss of consciousness leads to more atrophy.

Ng and colleagues[20] conducted a longitudinal study using structural MR imaging in 14 adults with moderate to severe TBI from an inpatient neurorehabilitation program and found subacute progression of brain atrophy, from 4.5 months to 29 months postinjury.

Wilde and colleagues[21] found significant volume loss in the hippocampus, amygdala, and globus pallidus, comparing 16 children with moderate to severe TBI in comparison with age-matched controls.

Cavum Septum and Ventricular Enlargement

The CSP describes a septum pellucidum that has a separation between its 2 leaflets (septal laminae). This cavity contains cerebrospinal fluid that filters from the ventricles through the septal laminae.[22] The cavum vergae is a posterior extension of the CSP. Although the CSP is believed to represent an anatomic variant,[23,24] an increased incidence has been reported in autopsy in patients with CTE.[4] Other investigators have reported an increased prevalence of CSP in sports players and military combatants (Figs. 1 and 2).

Comparing the high-resolution structural 3T MR imaging of 72 symptomatic former professional football players with 14 former professional noncontact sports athletes, Koerte and colleagues[25] found a higher rate of CSP (92% vs 57%) and a greater length of CSP as well as a greater ratio of CSP length to septum length in symptomatic former professional football players compared with athlete controls. In addition, a greater length of CSP was associated with decreased performance on a list learning task and decreased test scores on a measure of estimate verbal intelligence.

Lee and colleagues[26] analyzed the conventional 3T MR imaging findings in 499 fighters (boxers, mixed martial artists, and martial artists) and 62 controls for nonspecific white matter changes, cerebral microhemorrhage, CSP, and cavum vergae. The investigators found a significantly increased prevalence of CSP among fighters versus controls (53.1% vs 17.7%; $P<.001$). Although cerebral microhemorrhages were higher in fighters than in controls, this finding was not statistically significant, possibly partially due to underpowering of the study.

Gardner and colleagues[27] compared the CSP in patients presenting to a memory clinic, including 17 retired profootball players versus matched controls. The investigators found a higher prevalence (94% vs 3%) of CSP in retired profootball players compared with patients without a history of TBI.

Orrison and colleagues[28] found a cavum of the septum pellucidum in 43 of 100 unselected consecutive professional unarmed combatants who underwent brain MR imaging.

White Matter Changes

Strong evidence of structural changes in the white matter in patients with mTBI has been found in multiple imaging modalities.

Fluid-attenuated inversion recovery (FLAIR) changes in the white matter are common in patients with moderate and severe TMI but less frequent in patients with mTBI. Marquez de la Plata and colleagues[29] studied the white matter lesion volume visible in FLAIR in 24 patients with moderate to severe TBI without extra-axial or major cortical contusions and found a correlation

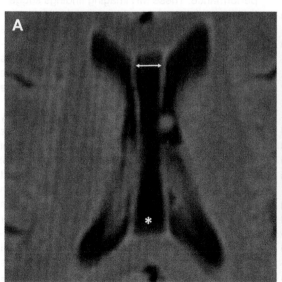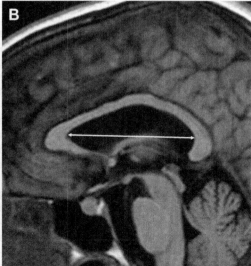

Fig. 1. Cavum of the septum pellucidum and cavum vergae. (A) Axial FLAIR demonstrates the width of a cavum of the septum pellucidum (arrow). A cavum vergae more posteriorly (asterisk) is demonstrated. (B) Sagittal T1-weighted imaging demonstrates the length of the cavum of the septum pellucidum (arrow).

between total diffuse axonal injury volume and unfavorable functional outcome 6 months after injury.

The white matter changes induced by TBI are not static. Johnson and colleagues[12] performed autopsy studies of 52 subjects who died from TBI and 44 age-matched controls from the Glasgow Traumatic Brain Injury Archive. This study found reactive microglia and reduction in the corpus callosum thickness with survival greater than 1 year postinjury. During the first year after moderate and severe TBI, Moen and colleagues[30] demonstrated a slowly evolving disruption of the microstructure in normal appearing corpus callosum in the apparent diffusion coefficient map, most evident in the posterior truncus. The mean apparent diffusion coefficient values were associated with both outcome and ability to perform speeded, complex sensory-motor action.

Hulkower and colleagues[31] performed a quantitative literature review of 100 articles reporting the use DTI to detect brain abnormalities in patients with TBI. Despite significant variability in sample characteristics, technical aspects of imaging, and analysis approaches, the consensus is that DTI effectively differentiates patients with TBI and controls, regardless of the severity and timeframe after injury. Furthermore, many have established a relationship between DTI measures and TBI outcomes. The heterogeneity of specific outcome measures, however, used limits interpretation of the literature. Similarly, few longitudinal studies have been performed, limiting inferences regarding the long-term predictive utility of DTI. Larger longitudinal studies, using standardized imaging, analysis approaches, and outcome measures, will help realize the promise of DTI as a prognostic tool in the care of patients with TBI. By far, fractional anisotropy was the DTI measure used most commonly across the studies the investigators reviewed. DTI, diffusion kurtosis imaging, and diffusion basis spectrum imaging are other MR imaging–based imaging modalities that demonstrate structural changes in the white matter.[7] Inglese and colleagues[32] studied a cohort of 46 patients with mTBI and 29 healthy volunteers using DTI and found subtle mean diffusivity and fractional anisotropy abnormalities in brain areas that are frequent sites of diffuse axonal injury.

Many studies of white matter changes are being conducted in populations of sports related concussion. Coughlin and colleagues[33] conducted a study in a cohort of National Football League (NFL) players and control participants, using PET-based regional measures of translocator protein 18 kDa, a marker of activated glial cell response; DTI measures of regional white matter integrity; regional volumes on structural MR imaging; and

neuropsychological performance. The investigators found higher translocator protein 18 kDa signal and white matter changes, which may be associated with NFL play.

Zhang and colleagues[34] compared the average diffusion constant of the entire brain and diffusion distribution width in 24 boxers and in 14 age-matched and gender-matched control subjects with no history of head trauma. This study showed that boxers had higher diffusion constants than those in control subjects. The investigators concluded that microstructural damage of the brain associated with chronic TBI may elevate whole-brain diffusion. This global elevation can exist even when routine MR findings are normal.

Lancaster and colleagues[35] studied the white matter changes within 24 hours of concussion and at 24 hours and 8 days postinjury in a group of high school and collegiate athletes, using DTI and diffusion kurtosis tensor imaging (DKTI) metrics. At 24 hours postinjury, the concussed group reported significantly more concussion symptoms than a well-matched control group and demonstrated poorer performance on a cognitive screening measure, yet these differences were nonsignificant at the 8-day follow-up. Similarly, within 24-hours after injury, the concussed group exhibited a widespread decrease in mean diffusivity, increased axial kurtosis, and, to a lesser extent, decreased axial and radial diffusivities compared with control subjects. At 8 days postinjury, the differences in these diffusion metrics were even more widespread in the injured athletes, despite improvement of symptoms and cognitive performance. These MR imaging findings suggest that the athletes might not have reached full physiologic recovery a week after the injury. These findings have significant implications for the management of sports related concussion because allowing an athlete to return to play before the brain has fully recovered from injury may have negative consequences.

Davenport and colleagues[36] conducted a study using DTI to examine white matter integrity, as quantified by fractional anisotropy, in a group of American military service members with (n = 25) or without (n = 33) blast-related mTBI. Blast mTBI was associated with a diffuse, global pattern of lower white matter integrity, and this pattern was not affected by previous civilian mTBI. Neither type of mTBI had an effect on the measures sensitive to more concentrated and spatially consistent white matter disruptions. Additionally, individuals with more than 1 blast mTBI tended to have a larger number of low fractional anisotropy voxels than individuals with a single blast injury. These results indicate that blast mTBI is associated with

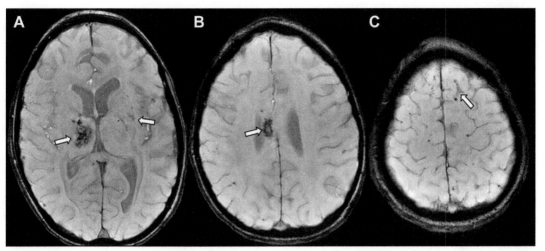

Fig. 2. Susceptibility weighted images in a patient with diffuse axonal injury demonstrate confluent microhemorrhages in multiple regions. (*A*) Right thalamus and left basal ganglia (*arrows*). (*B*) Corpus callosum (*arrow*). (*C*) Subcortical white matter (*arrow*).

disrupted integrity of several white matter tracts and that these disruptions are diluted by averaging across the large number of voxels within an ROI. The reported pattern of effects supports the conclusion that the neurologic effects of blast mTBI are diffuse, widespread, and spatially variable.

Microhemorrhages

Hähnel and colleagues[37] compared the presence of microhemorrhages in 42 male, classical amateur boxers and in 37 healthy, nonboxing male volunteers using brain MR imaging at 3T. Although the investigators detected more microhemorrhages in amateur boxers than in nonboxing persons, this difference did not prove significant. Similarly, Hasiloglu and colleagues[38] compared the prevalence of microhemorrhages in brain MR imaging at 1.5T in 21 amateur boxers versus 21 control subjects and did not find a statistically significant difference.

In a study of 499 fighters (boxers, mixed martial artists, and martial artists) and 62 controls, Lee and colleagues[26] found that fighters had a 4.2% prevalence of cerebral microhemorrhage (vs 0% for controls; $P = .152$). Although cerebral microhemorrhages were higher in fighters than in controls, this finding was not statistically significant, possibly partially due to underpowering of the study (**Fig. 2**).

FUTURE DIRECTIONS

Similar to other fields, the research of mTBI is limited by the heterogeneity of the imaging modalities, population selection, and the sample sizes. To address this limitation, multiple imaging repositories are being compiled. The NINDS-funded, multicenter Transforming Research and Clinical Knowledge in Traumatic Brain Injury (TRACK-TBI) study aims to collect and analyze detailed clinical data on 3000 subjects at 11 US sites, across the injury spectrum, along with CT/MR imaging, blood biospecimens, and detailed clinical outcomes. The TRACK-TBI pilot data set is the first to populate the Federal Interagency Traumatic Brain Injury Research (FITBIR) repository and with the current TRACK-TBI data is compatible with the International Initiative for Traumatic Brain Injury Research, a collaborative effort of the European Commission, the Canadian Institutes of Health Research, and the National Institutes of Health. The FITBIR Informatics System (https://fitbir.nih.gov/) is the result of a collaboration that began in 2011 between the National Institutes of Health and the US Department of Defense. Its purpose is to create a national resource for archiving and sharing clinical data from research studies on TBI, along with appropriate control data.[39]

REFERENCES

1. McCrory P, Meeuwisse WH, Aubry M, et al. Consensus statement on concussion in sport: the 4th international conference on concussion in sport, Zurich, November 2012. J Athl Train 2013;48: 554–75.
2. Esopenko C, Levine B. Aging, neurodegenerative disease, and traumatic brain injury: the role of neuroimaging. J Neurotrauma 2015;32:209–20.

3. Omalu BI, DeKosky ST, Hamilton RL, et al. Chronic traumatic encephalopathy in a National Football League player. Neurosurgery 2006;59(5):1086–92.

4. McKee AC, Stern RA, Nowinski CJ, et al. The spectrum of disease in chronic traumatic encephalopathy. Brain 2013;136:43–64.

5. McKee AC, Cairns NJ, Dickson DW, et al. The first NINDS/NIBIB consensus meeting to define neuropathological criteria for the diagnosis of chronic traumatic encephalopathy. Acta Neuropathol 2016; 131:75–86.

6. Giza CC, Hovda DA. The neurometabolic cascade of concussion. J Athl Train 2001;36:228–35.

7. Kou Z, VandeVord PJ. Traumatic white matter injury and glial activation: from basic science to clinics. Glia 2014;62:1831–55.

8. Chapman JC, Diaz-Arrastia R. Military traumatic brain injury: a review. Alzheimers Dement 2014;10: S97–104.

9. Gavett BE, Stern RA, Cantu RC, et al. Mild traumatic brain injury: a risk factor for neurodegeneration. Alzheimers Res Ther 2010;2:18.

10. Mez J, Stern RA, McKee AC. Chronic traumatic encephalopathy: where are we and where are we going? Curr Neurol Neurosci Rep 2013;13:407.

11. Washington PM, Villapol S, Burns MP. Polypathology and dementia after brain trauma: does brain injury trigger distinct neurodegenerative diseases, or should they be classified together as traumatic encephalopathy? Exp Neurol 2016; 275(Pt 3):381–8.

12. Johnson VE, Stewart JE, Begbie FD, et al. Inflammation and white matter degeneration persist for years after a single traumatic brain injury. Brain 2013;136: 28–42.

13. Jordan BD. The clinical spectrum of sport-related traumatic brain injury. Nat Rev Neurol 2013;9:222–30.

14. Koerte IK, Hufschmidt J, Muehlmann M, et al. A review of neuroimaging findings in repetitive brain trauma. Brain Pathol 2015;25:318–49.

15. Wintermark M, Sanelli PC, Anzai Y, et al. Imaging evidence and recommendations for traumatic brain injury: advanced neuro- and neurovascular imaging techniques. AJNR Am J Neuroradiol 2015;36:E1–11.

16. Smits M, Hunink MG, van Rijssel DA, et al. Outcome after complicated minor head injury. AJNR Am J Neuroradiol 2008;29:506–13.

17. Haacke EM, Duhaime AC, Gean AD, et al. Common data elements in radiologic imaging of traumatic brain injury. J Magn Reson Imaging 2010;32:516–43.

18. Ross DE. Review of longitudinal studies of MRI brain volumetry in patients with traumatic brain injury. Brain Inj 2011;25:1271–8.

19. MacKenzie JD, Siddiqi F, Babb JS, et al. Brain atrophy in mild or moderate traumatic brain injury: a longitudinal quantitative analysis. Am J Neuroradiol 2002;23:1509–15.

20. Ng K, Mikulis DJ, Glazer J, et al. Magnetic resonance imaging evidence of progression of subacute brain atrophy in moderate to severe traumatic brain injury. Arch Phys Med Rehabil 2008;89:S35–44.

21. Wilde EA, Bigler ED, Hunter JV, et al. Hippocampus, amygdala, and basal ganglia morphometrics in children after moderate-to-severe traumatic brain injury. Dev Med Child Neurol 2007;49:294–9.

22. Oteruelo FT. On the cavum septi pellucidi and the cavum Vergae. Anat Anz 1986;162:271–8.

23. Born CM, Meisenzahl EM, Frodl T, et al. The septum pellucidum and its variants. An MRI study. Eur Arch Psychiatry Clin Neurosci 2004;254:295–302.

24. Gur RE, Kaltman D, Melhem ER, et al. Incidental findings in youths volunteering for brain MRI research. Am J Neuroradiol 2013;34:2021–5.

25. Koerte I, Tripodis Y, Stamm JM, et al. Cavum septi pellucidi in symptomatic former professional football players. J Neurotrauma 2016;33(4):346–53.

26. Lee JK, Wu J, Banks S, et al. Prevalence of traumatic findings on routine MRI in a large cohort of professional fighters. Am J Neuroradiol 2017;38:1303–10.

27. Gardner RC, Hess CP, Brus-Ramer M, et al. Cavum septum pellucidum in retired american pro-football players. J Neurotrauma 2016;33:157–61.

28. Orrison WW, Hanson EH, Alamo T, et al. Traumatic brain injury: a review and high-field MRI findings in 100 unarmed combatants using a literature-based checklist approach. J Neurotrauma 2009;26: 689–701.

29. Marquez de la Plata C, Ardelean A, Koovakkattu D, et al. Magnetic resonance imaging of diffuse axonal injury: quantitative assessment of white matter lesion volume. J Neurotrauma 2007;24:591–8.

30. Moen KG, Håberg AK, Skandsen T, et al. A longitudinal magnetic resonance imaging study of the apparent diffusion coefficient values in corpus callosum during the first year after traumatic brain injury. J Neurotrauma 2013;31:56–63.

31. Hulkower MB, Poliak DB, Rosenbaum SB, et al. Decade of DTI in traumatic brain injury: 10 years and 100 articles later. Am J Neuroradiol 2013;34: 2064–74.

32. Inglese M, Makani S, Johnson G, et al. Diffuse axonal injury in mild traumatic brain injury: a diffusion tensor imaging study. J Neurosurg 2005;103: 298–303.

33. Coughlin JM, Wang Y, Minn I, et al. Imaging of glial cell activation and white matter integrity in brains of active and recently retired national football league players. JAMA Neurol 2017;74:67–74.

34. Zhang L, Ravdin LD, Relkin N, et al. Increased diffusion in the brain of professional boxers: a preclinical sign of traumatic brain injury? Am J Neuroradiol 2003;24:52–7.

35. Lancaster MA, Olson DV, McCrea MA, et al. Acute white matter changes following sport-related

concussion: a serial diffusion tensor and diffusion kurtosis tensor imaging study. Hum Brain Mapp 2016;37:3821–34.

36. Davenport ND, Lim KO, Armstrong MT, et al. Diffuse and spatially variable white matter disruptions are associated with blast-related mild traumatic brain injury. Neuroimage 2012;59:2017–24.

37. Hähnel S, Stippich C, Weber I, et al. Prevalence of cerebral microhemorrhages in amateur boxers as detected by 3T MR imaging. Am J Neuroradiol 2008;29:388–91.

38. Hasiloglu ZI, Albayram S, Selcuk H, et al. Cerebral microhemorrhages detected by susceptibility-weighted imaging in amateur boxers. AJNR Am J Neuroradiol 2011;32:99–102.

39. Wintermark M, Coombs L, Druzgal TJ, et al. Traumatic brain injury imaging research roadmap. Am J Neuroradiol 2015;36:E12–23.

Moving?

Make sure your subscription moves with you!

To notify us of your new address, find your **Clinics Account Number** (located on your mailing label above your name), and contact customer service at:

Email: journalscustomerservice-usa@elsevier.com

800-654-2452 (subscribers in the U.S. & Canada)
314-447-8871 (subscribers outside of the U.S. & Canada)

Fax number: 314-447-8029

Elsevier Health Sciences Division
Subscription Customer Service
3251 Riverport Lane
Maryland Heights, MO 63043

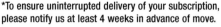

*To ensure uninterrupted delivery of your subscription, please notify us at least 4 weeks in advance of move.

ELSEVIER

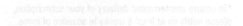

Printed and bound by CPI Group (UK) Ltd, Croydon, CR0 4YY

03/10/2024

01040304-0006